ABC OF VASCULAR DISEASES

ABC OF VASCULAR DISEASES

edited by

JOHN H N WOLFE FRCS

Consultant vascular surgeon, St Mary's Hospital, London

with contributions by

GEOFFREY ROSE, ANDREW N NICOLAIDES, D T REILLY, M A AL-KUTOUBI, G A D McPHERSON, N J W CHESHIRE, S J D CHADWICK, R S ELKELES, P R TAYLOR, AVERIL O MANSFIELD, SIMON R G SMITH, P RUTTER, N F G HOPKINS, JOHN T HOBBS, E L GILLILAND, M H GRIGG, D J THOMAS, D J ALLISON, ANNE KENNEDY

Articles published in
the *British Medical Journal*

Published by the British Medical Journal
Tavistock Square, London WC1H 9JR

First published 1992

British Library Cataloguing in Publication Data

ISBN 0–7279–0259–8

Printed in Great Britain by Jolly & Barber Ltd, Rugby
Typesetting by Bedford Typesetters Ltd, Bedford

Contents

FOREWORD

Vascular problems, so common in family and hospital practice, have long been their Cinderella, often forgotten and sometimes neglected. Yet we should all know the correct grade of elastic support, the importance of the different kinds of leg veins, the needs of obstinate ankle ulcers, the meaning and relief of numb fingers and lame leg muscles. Retirement marred by the obtrusion of an abdominal aneurysm; early warnings of a possible stroke; the catastrophe of an unheralded pulmonary embolism; all these and much more are presented in these pages. The St Mary's school of vascular surgery has produced clear practical messages and guidance, yet the basic mechanisms and research of promise are also covered. I congratulate the team on a much needed approach, avoiding the esoteric and keeping to reality. They have opened a new door to healing and relief for this large and sometimes overlooked population of patients.

H H G Eastcott

Former consultant vascular surgeon,
St Mary's Hospital

March 1992

INTRODUCTION

Alexis Carrel won a Nobel Prize in 1912 for his pioneering work in experimental vascular surgery. Since then the incidence of vascular diseases has reached epidemic proportions. The risks of infection prevented the widespread adoption of surgical treatment of patients until the advent of antibiotics, but in recent years there has been an exponential increase in the number of patients treated. This has been accompanied by the development of non-invasive methods of investigation; improvements in perioperative care; and better grafts, sutures, and instruments, as well as a plethora of new surgical and radiological procedures.

The successful treatment of vascular diseases now requires cooperation among many hospital specialists—vascular surgeons, general surgeons, radiologists, neurologists, cardiologists, orthopaedic surgeons, and general physicians—as well as among paramedical staff, physiotherapists, occupational therapists, and nurses from intensive care units, wards, and the community. One of the most important figures, however, is the general practitioner, who has a vital part to play throughout. This book attempts to draw the contributions of all these together in short, clear, chapters.

I am indebted to many colleagues for their contributions, which present a cohesive picture of the diagnosis and treatment of vascular diseases today. I thank the audiovisual department, St Mary's Hospital, London, for their help in the preparation of the illustrations, and finally I thank Alison des Landes and Pat Cairns for their continuing support and help with the preparation of the manuscript.

JOHN H N WOLFE

St Mary's Hospital,
London

March 1992

*This book is dedicated to my children, Tara, Robert, Roshean, Owen, and Matthew,
and to the stoical staff and patients of the Zachary Cope Ward, St Mary's Hospital, London*

EPIDEMIOLOGY OF ATHEROSCLEROSIS

Geoffrey Rose

The problem: its nature and scale

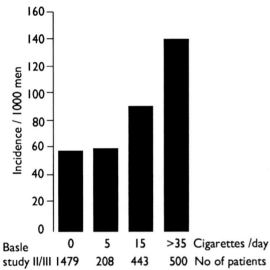

| Basle study II/III | 0 | 5 | 15 | >35 Cigarettes /day |
| | 1479 | 208 | 443 | 500 No of patients |

Five year incidence of peripheral arterial occlusive disease according to how many cigarettes smoked, from the Basle study.

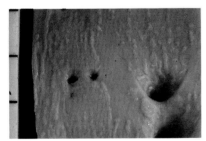

Fatty streaks—the early development of atheroma in areas of low shear stress around ostia.

Most diseases affect only an unfortunate minority, but in Britain few people reach "old age" without a potentially dangerous degree of atherosclerosis. Half of all deaths are caused by circulatory diseases, and over 40% of middle aged men have evidence of ischaemia that is the result of atherosclerosis.

Lipid streaks begin to appear in the aortic intima before the age of 10, but these are not important. Real atherosclerosis starts during the teens and in early life it spreads rapidly. By itself it causes little trouble; increasingly, however, the plaques cause fissures and haemorrhages, which in turn may lead to thrombosis (particularly in the carotid arteries) embolisation and consequent ischaemia.

Often the first clinical event is dramatic—a stroke or sudden death (the first presentation of coronary heart disease in 20% of cases); even in non-fatal presentations there is usually much irreversible disease. The real course of atherosclerotic disease, however, is usually extremely slow, the serious event usually being preceded—years in advance—by small signs of developing ischaemia. For example, only a few people with angina or intermittent claudication actually attend the doctor and are diagnosed. Minor disease usually goes unrecognised but when it is recognised it is the best predictor of future serious disease.

Atherosclerosis is always a more or less generalised—albeit patchy—condition. The patient with intermittent claudication will probably die of a coronary thrombosis, and the surgeon who relieves coronary stenosis needs to remember that the patient still has generalised arterial disease.

The same underlying causes and risk factors are found no matter at what site the problem presents. People with hypercholesterolaemia or hypertension get more of the same sort of atherosclerosis and the pathologist cannot tell one from another. The clinical consequences are, however, extremely varied, and similar clinical syndromes may be caused by non-atherosclerotic disease.

For reasons that we do not understand men are much more prone than women to almost all forms of vascular disease (especially aortic aneurysms). Women's protection wanes gradually with age, and by "old age" the risks are similar for the two sexes. At any age the protection is wiped out by diabetes.

Underlying causes

Mortality from coronary disease in the United States has fallen by 40% in less than 20 years

Arterial disease is not—as we used to be taught—degenerative (except for the loss of elasticity in larger arteries and veins that is associated with age). In some remote societies it is uncommon even in old age. Nor is it a necessary accompaniment of twentieth century affluence: mortality from coronary disease is low and falling, and in the United States has fallen by 40% in less than 20 years. In Britain mortality from coronary disease among manual workers continues to rise, but among other groups it is now falling; clearly the incidence of arterial disease is at least potentially reducible.

Epidemiology of atherosclerosis

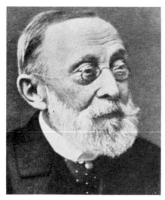

Rudolf Virchow, whose triad of the causes of thrombosis remains valid today: disease of the wall, consistency of the blood, and abnormality of the flow.

Who is at risk?

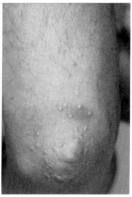

Self mutilation by smoking—this patient had all four limbs amputated for a Buerger's type of arteritis. His cigarette holder was made out of a coat hanger by one of his friends on the ward.

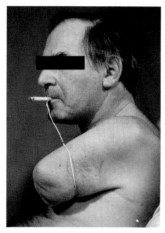

Xanthomas on the elbow.

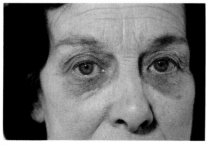

Xanthelasma.

The one essential underlying cause of serious atherosclerosis seems to be a high concentration of low density lipoprotein in the blood, which reflects a high intake of dietary saturated fat. The Japanese do not have this and so—despite a high incidence of smoking and hypertension—they have fewer atherosclerotic problems. When the concentration of low density lipoprotein is high, however, other factors may aggravate the process. In particular, the enormous variation in incidence seems to depend on the number of smokers and patients with diabetes or high blood pressure in the particular community (the last two reflecting overweight).

Large pieces of this jigsaw remain to be discovered. Probably some key pieces concern the regulators of thrombosis. Thus men in Edinburgh have twice the incidence of coronary disease as their Stockholm contemporaries despite similar "classic" risk factors. The explanation may be that they have a much lower intake of linoleic acid, a fatty acid essential for prostaglandin synthesis and possibly an important determinant of platelet and endothelial stickiness. Atherosclerosis may be the precursor of ischaemia but thrombosis is commonly the precipitator.

The simple answer is that everyone is at risk, but some much more than others. Even those in the lowest risk category are more likely to die of cardiovascular disease than of any other single cause, but they will get the disease later in life. The same risk factors apply to all the main forms of arterial disease but the balance is different. Stroke is dominated by blood pressure, whereas diabetes and smoking are most strongly linked with ischaemia of the legs.

Clues from the patient's background come from:

● Residence—south west Scotland and northern Ireland have the highest incidences

● Occupation—the rates are highest, and still rising, among manual and unskilled workers, and

● Family history—but only if the relatives developed the disease before the age of 60.

Serum low density lipoprotein concentration

The first of the three main personal risk factors is the serum concentration of low density lipoprotein. Total cholesterol concentration is, however, an adequate guide and its measurement does not require fasting. The laboratory's so called "reference range" should be ignored; it refers only to what is common and not to what is advisable. Recent evidence makes it clear that there is no threshold of risk. The average serum cholesterol concentration in middle age is about 6·3 mmol/l, but biologically this is high and the ideal is somewhere under 5 mmol/l. More heart attacks occur in patients with average or above average cholesterol concentrations (because they are so numerous) than among the small minority with conspicuous hypercholesterolaemia. This minority, however, do need special help. Blood cholesterol screening should be selective and measurement of high density lipoproteins and triglycerides does not add much to the basic assessment of risk if other risk factors are already known.

Blood pressure

As a guide to risk systolic blood pressure is as valid as the diastolic measurement, and the initial measurement can be regarded as predictive. As a guide to treatment, however, multiple checks at several visits are needed. Risk is graded, as for cholesterol measurement, and most vascular disease is associated with mild hypertension because it is so common. The risk of stroke reflects current blood pressure, and it is swiftly reversed by treatment. For reasons that we do not understand the same is not true of the risk of coronary thrombosis; this is less affected by antihypertensive drugs and we must control other risk factors to reduce it.

Risk factors for atherosclerosis

- Smoking

- Blood pressure

- Diet

- Diabetes

- Blood cholesterol concentration

The risk of heart attack is trebled if the patient smokes, has a serum cholesterol concentration of 6 mmol/l, *and* has a diastolic blood pressure of 85 mm Hg

---

Treatment of arterial disease

- Operation

- Control of hypertension, blood sugar, and lipids

- Thrombolytic drugs

- **STOP SMOKING**

Smoking

The third important risk factor is smoking—especially cigarettes but probably also pipes and cigars if the smoke is inhaled. Smoking roughly doubles the risk of heart attack and (in hypertensive patients) of stroke, and it massively aggravates the progression of ischaemic complications of peripheral arterial disease. The number of cigarettes smoked seems less important than the mere fact of smoking, and the type of cigarette is largely irrelevant (for the vascular system there is no "safer cigarette"). Unfortunately we still do not know the guilty component(s) of tobacco smoke or their mode of action, but this probably includes thrombogenesis, and stopping smoking brings swift benefit.

Combinations of risk factors

Combinations of risk factors are the main trouble makers. The risk of coronary disease is roughly trebled by a serum cholesterol concentration of 9 mmol/l or by a diastolic blood pressure of 115 mm Hg, and when seen these will not be overlooked because they are most unusual. The risk is also trebled (compared with a low risk subject) by cigarette smoking, plus a cholesterol concentration of 6 mmol/l, plus a diastolic pressure of 85 mm Hg—a combination so common that the doctor may say "My patient has no risk factors." Most vascular disease is caused by such combinations because the arteries stand up reasonably well to one single factor in isolation. The therapeutic corollary of this is that management must also take account of all aspects. Surgery, acute care of patients with myocardial infarction, control of blood sugar concentrations in diabetes, or control of blood pressure in hypertension—each is just one component in the management of a chronic disease with many causes.

The data from the Basle study were presented by Schering. The pictures of self mutilation by smoking and the fatty streaks are reproduced by kind permission of Professor Sir Geoffrey Slaney, KBE, FRCS, and Professor Neville Woolf, PHD, FRCPATH, respectively.

ASSESSMENT OF LEG ISCHAEMIA

Andrew N Nicolaides

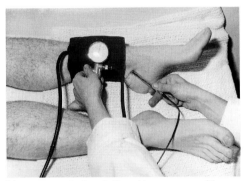

Measurement of systolic ankle pressure with simple inexpensive equipment: pneumatic cuff and pressure gauge (left), and Doppler ultrasound velocimeter (right) to detect dorsalis pedis and posterior tibial signals.

Pain on walking is a common complaint usually caused by arthritis or sciatica, but stenosis of the spinal canal and venous insufficiency must also be considered before ischaemia is confirmed. This is easy in most patients, but may be difficult if the ischaemia is mild, or there is coexistent arthritis. Evidence of peripheral ischaemia such as skin changes, cold feet, and absent pulses will confirm any suspicion of arterial disease that has been raised by the history. Rest pain, especially at night, is diagnostic, and urgent admission to hospital for arteriography should be arranged with the expectation of early operation for revascularisation. In some claudicant patients, however, there may not be such clear cut evidence of ischaemia because there are no skin changes and all the peripheral pulses are present when the patient is examined at rest.

Patients can be divided into four main groups:

● Those in whom femoral pulses are absent or weak, suggesting the presence of aortoiliac disease

● Those with absent foot pulses but normal femoral pulses, suggesting femorodistal disease

● Those whose foot and femoral pulses are normal at rest but become weak or disappear on exercise

● Those with normal foot and femoral pulses at rest that are not altered by exercise.

Most patients can be diagnosed by simple and careful history taking and examination. Decisions about treatment, while based on the clinical features above, may be clarified by non-invasive investigations. In most patients arteriography can be avoided.

Is there arterial disease?

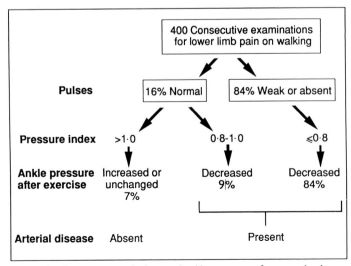

Value of pulses, pressure index, and ankle pressure after exercise in determining the presence or absence of arterial disease.

If the pulses are absent the clinical examination alone is enough to determine the presence of arterial disease; non-invasive tests are not necessary to make the diagnosis and they are used mainly to document the presence and extent of disease. If the pulses are weak the non-invasive tests are also unnecessary but they can provide objective quantitative confirmation. The ankle pressure at rest is simple to measure, confirms the clinical impression, and is particularly useful in obese patients or if there is ankle oedema that makes the pulses difficult to feel. If the pulses are normal, however, and the patient has pain on walking, further tests are necessary. In such patients the ankle pressure should be measured both at rest and after exercise because it is possible to have normal ankle pressures at rest, and a fall in ankle pressure after exercise may be the sole indicator of disease.

A fall in ankle pressure after a standardised exercise test on a treadmill is the most sensitive measure of the presence of occlusive arterial disease. A study of 400 patients with pain on walking showed the comparative accuracy of assessment of the pulses and measurement of the pressure indexes at rest and the ankle pressures after exercise. The ankle pressure after exercise was the most sensitive index of the presence of severe disease, and relying on the pulses alone would have resulted in the wrong diagnosis in 9% of patients. Whenever the ankle pressure after exercise was increased or unchanged the aortogram was normal and the symptoms were the result of other conditions such as osteoarthritis, sciatica, or venous insufficiency. Thus if there was an increase in ankle pressure after exercise severe arterial disease could be excluded and patients spared unnecessary investigations.

> The ankle pressure after exercise is the most sensitive sign of the presence of arterial disease

How severe is the disease?

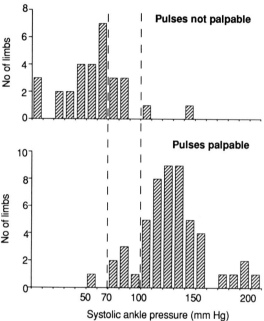

Relation of ankle pressure to presence or absence of foot pulses in a study of 82 limbs.

From the history and clinical examination patients may be divided into three groups:

- Those with mild disease and mild claudication
- Those with moderate disease and severe claudication
- Those with disease so severe that the limb is in danger.

The measurement of ankle pressures was simplified in the late 1960s when instruments were developed that could detect flow in small vessels distal to a pneumatic cuff. The grading of pulses by palpation as normal, weak, or absent lacks precision, however sensitive the examiner's fingers may be.

When the ankle systolic pressure is 110 mm Hg foot pulses may be graded as normal, although this pressure may be only 60% of the brachial systolic pressure (180 mm Hg) in a patient with claudication. At a pressure of 70 mm Hg the foot is not in immediate danger, but at a pressure of 30 mm Hg it is, yet palpation may indicate absent pulses in both cases.

The decrease in ankle pressure after a standard exercise test and the time taken for it to return to the value before exercise (the recovery time) are good indicators of the severity of the disease, whereas the time of onset of claudication is an accurate measure of the patient's incapacity; this bears little relation to the patient's own assessment of his or her claudication distance. If the patient is tested after walking on the treadmill for one minute the test is simple, not unduly gruelling, and can be used to monitor the progression of the disease.

Where is the disease?

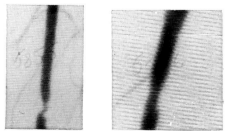

Arteriograms showing a severe stenosis of superficial femoral artery (left), and, immediately after balloon angioplasty, some residual stenosis (right).

There are good reasons for wanting to know whether the disease is in the aortoiliac segment, in the femoropopliteal segment, distal to the popliteal artery, or in more than one segment. In the case of aortoiliac reconstruction or percutaneous balloon angioplasty the results are good and the vessel may remain patent for many years, so that the patient remains free of symptoms. The results of femoropopliteal reconstruction, however, are not good; the primary failure rate is roughly 5-10% and between a third and a half of the grafts occlude within five years. Finally, attempts to reconstruct lesions distal to the popliteal artery are made only if the leg is critically ischaemic. Often the surgeon cannot decide by clinical observation alone whether there is also aortoiliac disease in a patient who has an obvious superficial femoral occlusion and palpable femoral pulses. Simple auscultation may show a bruit at the common femoral artery, but its importance may be difficult to assess.

A clue to the extent of disease can be obtained from the recovery time (the time taken for the decreased ankle pressure after exercise to return to the value before exercise). A recovery time of less than five minutes means that there is only a single lesion, and that it is most probably in the

Assessment of leg ischaemia

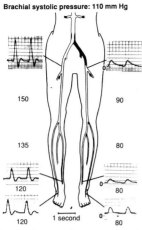

Brachial systolic pressure: 110 mm Hg

Blood velocity waveforms and systolic pressure in the lower limb in a patient with occlusion of the left iliac artery. Waveforms recorded from the common femoral, posterior tibial, and dorsalis pedis arteries are monophasic with identical acceleration and deceleration in all arteries.

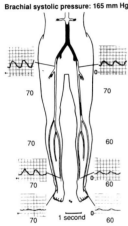

Brachial systolic pressure: 165 mm Hg

Waveforms recorded from the common femoral and posterior tibial arteries are different because of two segment disease.

femoropopliteal segment. A recovery time between 5 and 15 minutes also suggests a single lesion, but this is usually in the aortoiliac region. A recovery time of longer than 15 minutes suggests multiple lesions.

The recordings of Doppler velocity tracings from the common femoral artery together with velocity tracings from the ankle and the measurements made from them will supplement the pressure measurements and recovery time, and help to localise the disease because the velocity tracings distal to the stenosis or occlusion are dampened.

Is the aortoiliac segment normal?

The condition of the aortoiliac segment is fundamental in the management of claudication. After identifying the presence of occlusive arterial disease the surgeon should determine whether the aortoiliac segment is normal—that is, whether the disease is confined to the superficial femoral artery—because disease confined to the superficial femoral artery is a benign condition. I have found that about 92% of patients with superficial femoral artery occlusions whose aortoiliac segments are either normal or have less than 30% stenoses show spontaneous clinical improvement with improvement in ankle pressure readings.

How important is an aortoiliac lesion in patients with combined aortoiliac and femoropopliteal disease?

The femoral pulse and presence of a bruit may suggest aortoiliac disease. If the Doppler velocity tracings from the common femoral artery are triphasic, however, it means that the aortoiliac segment is normal.

The importance of disease in the aortoiliac segment in patients who require a femorodistal reconstruction is difficult to assess. Wave form analysis is useful and duplex assessment (Doppler and ultrasonographic imaging) of the aortoiliac segment may show localised stenoses. Many surgeons rely on the response of the femoral arterial pressure to dilatation of the distal arterial bed with 30 mg of papaverine. Providing that aortoiliac flow is adequate there is enough compensation for the increased requirement, but if there is proximal stenosis the injection of papaverine results in a decrease in pressure of 20 mm Hg or more in the femoral artery as the distal vascular bed expands.

The advent of duplex ultrasonic scanning with colour flow imaging has provided us with the ability to localise and grade the severity and extent of superficial femoral artery stenosis or occlusion. It is now possible to decide on the basis of this non-invasive scanning whether the lesion is suitable for balloon angioplasty without angiography.

Is there other important vascular disease?

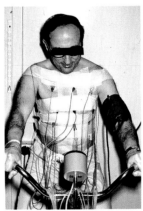

Patient exercising on a bicycle ergometer.

At least three quarters of patients presenting with peripheral arterial disease are likely to have serious vascular lesions elsewhere as well

Whether the surgeon recommends an operation depends on the severity of symptoms, the patient's incapacity, and the danger to the limb if the operation is not done, balanced against the risk of reconstruction and both the long term and the short term results. Surgeons must be able to estimate how long the reconstruction will last, and, finally, be able to say what the short term results will be. A patient will not be grateful for a successful arterial reconstruction if he or she is still incapacitated by angina or pain from an osteoarthritic hip. The surgeon must assess the severity of these conditions and decide whether their symptoms can be relieved too, as they commonly coexist with peripheral arterial disease. He or she may decide—for example—that a patient should have a coronary artery reconstruction and then peripheral arterial reconstruction.

Many patients with lower limb ischaemia have occult myocardial ischaemia. They give histories of one or more myocardial infarctions, or of angina that disappeared when their claudication distances decreased. In my experience over half the patients with claudication have electrocardiographic evidence of myocardial ischaemia on exercise, although only 3% develop angina. I have found that although their walking ability may be limited, they can exercise on a bicycle ergometer and raise their heart rates enough to give meaningful electrocardiographic results. In addition, the ability to diagnose the presence of one, two, or three vessel coronary disease by electrocardiographic chest wall mapping during bicycle ergometry offers the chance to select the high risk group that is responsible for the operative mortality (3-5%) and late mortality, which can be as high as 30% at two years.

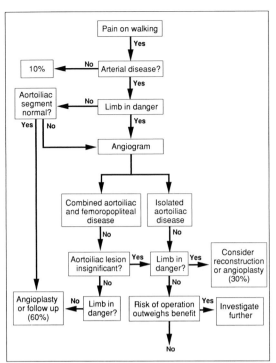

Initial management of patients with suspected arterial disease with decisions based on history, clinical examination, and information from non-invasive tests.

Further support for this comes from the Cleveland Clinic, where in a series of 1000 consecutive patients the presence of occult coronary disease was detected by routine coronary angiography in a large proportion of patients. The five year survival of patients with peripheral arterial disease and cardiac disease was 43% in the presence of severe three vessel coronary disease and 85% in the absence of such disease. Of those patients who had their severe coronary vessel disease corrected, however, 72% survived. Because of these figures a mortality of 20-40% at three years in patients with peripheral arterial disease is no longer acceptable. Referral of a patient for peripheral vascular reconstructive surgery provides an ideal opportunity for the diagnosis of associated coronary artery disease; such an opportunity may never occur again in his or her lifetime."

The questions posed by the physician and the clinical decisions that are based on the answers can be summarised by an algorithm. In my experience 10% of patients who attend because of pain on walking do not have arterial disease. I also find that 60% of the patients have mild claudication with superficial femoral occlusion and a normal iliac segment. These are treated conservatively. Thus 70% of patients are spared any further investigation and only 30% require an arteriogram.

Conclusion

Non-invasive tests permit:

- Confident exclusion of arterial disease
- Assessment of the affected segment
- Objective evidence of severity of disease

In summary, non-invasive tests are valuable adjuncts to the history and clinical examination. They permit confident exclusion of arterial disease, assessment of the affected segment, and objective evidence of the severity of disease. Finally, objective measurements of the progression of the disease and the follow up of reconstructions can be monitored.

The diagrams of blood velocity wave forms and systolic pressures are reproduced by kind permission of Churchill Livingstone.

THE YOUNG PATIENT WITH CLAUDICATION

D T Reilly, John H N Wolfe

> ### Causes of intermittent claudication
>
> - Atherosclerosis
> - Thromboembolism
> - Buerger's disease
> - Arteritis:
>   Systemic lupus erythematosus
>   Takayasu's disease
> - Fibrosis:
>   Retroperitoneal
>   Radiation
> - Developmental anomalies:
>   Coarctation
>   Persistent sciatic artery
>   Popliteal entrapment
> - Trauma
> - Cystic adventitial disease

All patients with intermittent claudication merit careful assessment, but the young claudicant patient in particular has much to gain from investigation, not only because an easily treatable lesion may be found but also because the long term outlook may be improved if risk factors are recognised and treated.

Most patients with intermittent claudication present at between 55 and 60 years of age, when the commonest cause is progression of atherosclerosis. In younger patients the other causes of claudication are proportionally more common. In this article we consider the patient who presents under the age of 50.

A conservative approach is often appropriate for the older claudicant patient, particularly if clinical examination suggests a superficial femoral artery occlusion. Exercise, giving up smoking, and changes in the diet can be effective, and the natural history of intermittent claudication is that only about a quarter of patients continue to deteriorate. This conservative course is not appropriate for the young claudicant patient, in whom the symptoms more dramatically affect lifestyle, unusual diagnoses assume greater importance, and thorough investigation of the arterial system should be encouraged. Extensive non-invasive investigation is now possible and less invasive methods of treatment are more accepted.

Diagnosis

> ### Risk factors in the atherosclerotic claudicant
>
> - Smoking
> - Diabetes mellitus
> - Hypertension
> - Hyperlipoproteinaemia
> - Renal disease
> - Family history of atherosclerosis

It is easy to overlook the symptoms in a 20 year old patient unless the possibility of intermittent claudication is kept in mind. There are, however, several possible causes of true intermittent claudication in a young person, including popliteal entrapment, cystic adventitial disease, and developmental anomalies. Venous claudication should not be overlooked in the differential diagnosis: there is the typical "bursting" sensation after walking that is relieved by raising the leg, and there is usually a history of injury or deep vein thrombosis. Atherosclerosis is common under the age of 50, particularly among heavy smokers, but the diagnosis of atherosclerosis as the principal cause of symptoms in this age group should lead to a search for risk factors and associated disease; there may well be a history of angina or transient ischaemic attacks. Atherosclerotic claudication may later lead to stroke, myocardial infarction, and possibly loss of a limb. In younger patients atherosclerosis pursues a more aggressive course than in older ones, so every attempt should be made to improve prognosis. The overall five year mortality for patients who present with intermittent claudication is about 30%.

Examination and investigation

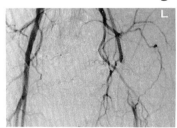

Dissection of left iliac artery causing unexpected claudication in a 34 year old man.

The clinical examination should pay particular attention to the presence of pulses, bruits, and signs of peripheral ischaemia. Aneurysms should be sought by careful palpation of the abdomen and the popliteal fossa; if a popliteal aneurysm is suspected it must be confirmed and treated because of the insidious embolisation of the distal run off vessels that occurs. By the time a popliteal aneurysm gives symptoms it may be too late for reconstruction.

The general examination should include careful cardiovascular evaluation, and orthopaedic examination may elicit or eliminate sciatica, spinal stenosis, and arthritis as causes of leg pain.

Specific conditions

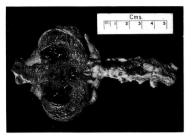

Histological specimen of thrombosed popliteal aneurysm.

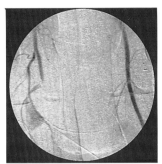

Digital subtraction arteriogram of popliteal entrapment on the right.

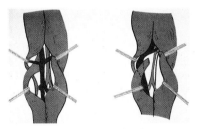

Normal popliteal artery (left) and popliteal entrapment (right).

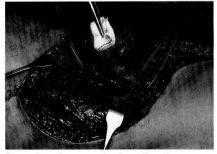

Operative photograph of popliteal aneurysm.

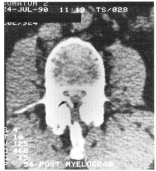

Spinal stenosis.

Popliteal aneurysm

The commonest cause of popliteal aneurysm is atherosclerosis, but other causes are popliteal artery entrapment, Marfan syndrome, and Ehlers-Danlos syndrome.

Atherosclerotic aneurysm—This is less common in the popliteal region than in the abdominal aorta, but 10% of patients with an abdominal aneurysm also have a popliteal aneurysm. Clinical suspicion is confirmed by ultrasound scanning, and arteriography should be carried out before operation, which entails ligation of the aneurysm together with vein or synthetic bypass grafting.

Popliteal entrapment—The underlying lesion is an abnormal origin of the gastrocnemius, usually the medial head, which compresses the artery and causes the intermittent claudication. On clinical examination the pulses may be normal, but it may be possible to make the foot pulses disappear by holding the leg in full extension with plantar flexion or dorsiflexion of the foot. If left untreated the compressed artery may become occluded with thrombus or develop a poststenotic aneurysm. Arteriography of both legs should be done because the condition is often bilateral. At operation the aberrant muscle bundle is simply divided and—if the artery is occluded or aneurysmal—an end to end vein graft interposed.

Other causes of popliteal aneurysm—Patients with Marfan syndrome are usually tall, and have other typical features including arachnodactyly, high arched palate, and dislocated lenses, and as a rule do not present with claudication. This is also true of patients with the Ehlers-Danlos syndrome, who have hyperextensible joints and hyperelastic skin. Patients with mycotic aneurysms are unlikely to present with claudication, but may present with fever, malaise, and local pain.

Other developmental anomalies

Coarctation of the aorta may present in a young patient as bilateral intermittent claudication, but more usually presents as hypertension. Femoral pulses are absent or diminished, and collateral vessels may easily be found on the chest wall. A persistent sciatic artery is a rare cause of intermittent claudication in a young person, and can be diagnosed only by arteriography; on clinical examination the popliteal and foot pulses are absent.

Cystic adventitial disease

Cystic adventitial disease is an uncommon condition of unknown aetiology in which the lumen of the popliteal artery is compressed by a cyst (similar to a ganglion) developing in the tunica media. Onset of claudication is abrupt because of rupture of the cyst or haemorrhage within it. A characteristic curved indentation of the lumen is seen on arteriography (the "scimitar" sign). Duplex Doppler scanning also shows the cysts and is probably the best investigation. Percutaneous transluminal angioplasty is of no use because the lesion is outside the intima; the choice of treatment is either operation (with excision of the cystic area and vein grafting if necessary), or the more recently advocated percutaneous puncture and drainage under computed tomographic control.

Trauma

Most patients with vascular trauma present acutely and require urgent revascularisation; delayed presentation with vascular insufficiency may occur, however, after recovery from a major limb fracture that caused intimal damage. Even if the pulses are palpable, measurement of ankle pressures helps to confirm or exclude a serious problem if the patient has intermittent claudication. In a young person reconstructive surgery with an interposition graft is likely to be well worth while.

Arteritis

Patients with arteritis who present with claudication usually have other symptoms. The typical patient with Buerger's disease is a man aged 30 to 40 who smokes heavily and has signs of advanced peripheral ischaemia and sometimes early distal ulceration or gangrene; there may also be associated thrombophlebitis. Systemic conditions associated with arteritis should be sought, such as systemic lupus erythematosus, scleroderma, and rheumatoid arthritis. Takayasu's disease is uncommon and was originally described in young Oriental women. It also occurs in European races and is

The young patient with claudication

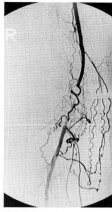

Right superficial femoral artery occlusion.

Investigations

General investigations
- Full blood count
- Erythrocyte sedimentation rate
- Serum concentrations of:
  Glucose
  Lipoproteins
  Triglycerides
  Urea
  Electrolytes
- Analysis of urine
- Chest radiography
- Electrocardiography

Special investigations
- Doppler ankle pressures
- Treadmill test
- Duplex Doppler ultrasound examination
- Arteriography:
  Digital
  Conventional

Management

Patients with absent femoral pulses are readily treatable

---

an arteritis principally affecting the vessels of the aortic arch, but it can also cause occlusion of the aortoiliac segment. The main features are an unusual distribution of arterial stenoses or occlusions in a young patient and the finding of a high erythrocyte sedimentation rate on investigation. The arteritis is treated with steroids, and the patient must stop smoking. The 10 year survival for Takayasu's disease without operation is about 90%.

Other causes of vascular insufficiency

Other causes of vascular insufficiency include such rarities as retroperitoneal fibrosis, which may be drug induced, idiopathic, or associated with granulomatous or malignant diseases. Aortoiliac stenosis can be caused by retroperitoneal fibrosis, in which case the clue will be diminished femoral pulses; standard bypass grafting should achieve a satisfactory result. Radiation fibrosis may also cause iliac occlusion, but is unlikely to be present in patients under 50 because of the long lag phase before radiation damage becomes apparent.

The most useful bedside test is the measurement of ankle pressures by Doppler ultrasonography. Hand held Doppler flow detectors cost about £300 and should be available in all surgical clinics. If the ankle pressures are normal when the patient is at rest the measurements can be repeated after standardised exercise on a treadmill. If the ratio of ankle pressure to brachial pressure does not fall, a haemodynamically important arterial lesion may be excluded.

Further evaluation of vascular lesions is now less invasive than formerly in centres equipped with facilities for digital vascular imaging and duplex Doppler scanning; for the younger and otherwise fit claudicant patient an arteriogram is nevertheless indicated to establish a firm diagnosis and to see whether there is a superficial femoral artery lesion that is amenable to percutaneous transluminal angioplasty. A further indication for arteriography (rather than a "wait and see" policy) is if the patient has weak femoral pulses and symptoms of aortoiliac disease such as buttock or thigh claudication and erectile impotence. These patients do not usually improve with time, whereas with a superficial femoral artery occlusion the claudication distance may increase considerably as collateral vessels develop. Furthermore, percutaneous angioplasty and surgery are extremely successful in the aortoilial segment.

General investigation of the atherosclerotic patient should include an exercise stress electrocardiogram, and a chest radiograph is important because most of these patients are smokers. Routine blood tests should include a full blood count (to detect polycythaemia or thrombocythaemia) and measurement of the erythrocyte sedimentation rate (to confirm arteritis), of urea and electrolyte concentrations—together with analysis of the urine—(to detect occult renal disease, of the blood glucose concentration (to detect diabetes mellitus), and of fasting lipoprotein and triglyceride concentrations (to diagnose hyperlipoproteinaemia). Tests for arteritis include measurement of antinuclear factor, DNA binding, rheumatoid factor, immunoglobulin, ANCA, SL70, cold agglutinin, and cryoglobulin concentrations. If the history suggests embolisation, with a sudden onset of symptoms in a patient with an otherwise normal vascular tree, an echocardiogram is indicated to search for the sourse of the emboli. When no obvious cause for the occlusion in apparent primary thrombosis may have occurred as a result of antithrombin III, protein C, or protein 5 deficiency. Homocystinuria may also predispose to thrombosis.

General

In the young atherosclerotic smoker the most important measures are to stop smoking, increase exercise, and change the diet. There is evidence that these are of long term benefit rather than punitive.

Though control of blood pressure and lipid concentrations may not be of such definite benefit to elderly people, there is increasing evidence that younger patients benefit from antihypertensive measures, dietary manipulation, and drugs to lower lipid concentrations such as cholestyramine (for hypercholesterolaemia), bezafibrate (for hypertriglyceridaemia), and gemfibrozil (for hyperlipidaemia).

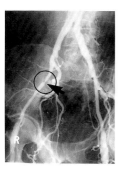

Stenosis of iliac artery (treatable).

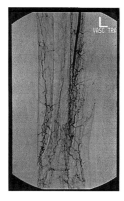

Buerger's disease (not treatable).

Specific measures in the atherosclerotic patient

Though great claims are made for drugs to improve blood flow or tissue metabolism, none has so far been shown to produce a convincing and clinically useful effect.

The introduction of percutaneous transluminal angioplasty greatly improved the treatment of occlusive vascular disease, but at the cost of an increased number of arteriograms. This is partly offset by the increased use of intravenous digital vascular imaging, which—though less invasive—still requires a large dose of contrast medium. It does not, however, require admission to hospital. Percutaneous transluminal angioplasty is effective in treating short stenoses or occlusions of both iliac and femoral arteries, and requires an overnight stay in hospital because of the size of the arterial puncture.

If the lesion is not amenable to transluminal angioplasty, surgery has to be considered. This will depend on the severity of the patient's symptoms, his or her general condition, and the extent and location of the disease. Bypass grafting in the leg is usually reserved for more severe ischaemia because of the decrease in patency in the long term and the small but real risk of endangering the limb. A patient who is unsuitable for percutaneous transluminal angioplasty and is affected by only moderate claudication without severe ischaemia may have to come to terms with his or her disease.

PERCUTANEOUS TRANSLUMINAL ANGIOPLASTY

M A Al-Kutoubi

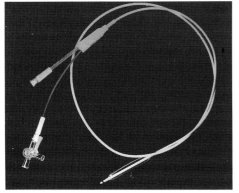

Balloon dilatation catheter.

Transluminal angioplasty was first described by Dotter and Judkins in 1964. They used coaxial catheters, but the technical limitations prevented its widespread acceptance until Gruntzig introduced the double lumen balloon catheter in 1976. This was both effective and easy to use, and established angioplasty as an acceptable technique for the treatment of vascular stenoses in most large arteries in the body. The simplicity and low associated morbidity have subtly altered the indications for intervention, but full clinical assessment of the patient and discussion with a vascular surgeon are essential before angioplasty is considered. There is no place for direct referral from a physician to a radiologist without consultation with a surgeon.

Mechanism of dilatation

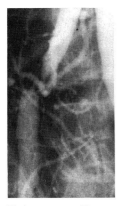
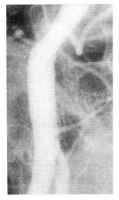

Right common iliac stenosis before (left) and after (right) balloon dilatation.

The stretching of the artery splits the intima, cracks the atheromatous plaques, and stretches—and sometimes ruptures—the media, causing local dissection and subintimal haemorrhage. Healing occurs by fibrosis and giant cell reaction with formation of neointima, resulting in a smooth lumen within a few weeks.

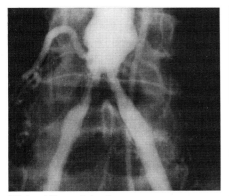

Bilateral iliac origin stenoses.

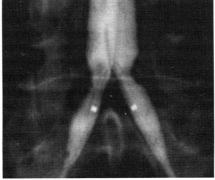

Bilateral iliac origin stenoses with "kissing" balloons in place.

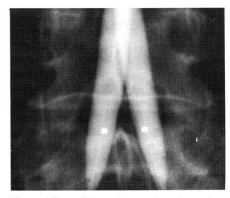

Bilateral iliac origin stenoses after plaque has been dilated.

Angioplasty of peripheral arteries

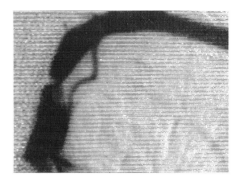

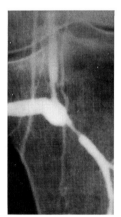

Left subclavian stenosis before (top) and after (bottom) balloon dilatation.

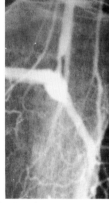

Stenosis at lower end of below knee femoropopliteal vein graft one year after operation before (left) and after (right) balloon dilatation.

Percutaneous transluminal angioplasty has been successfully used for the treatment of stenoses of the aorta and iliac, femoral, popliteal, and subclavian arteries; for treatment of stenosed grafts and arteriovenous dialysis shunts; as well as for stenoses of renal and mesenteric vessels and coronary arteries. Short occlusions of the femoropopliteal segment can be recanalised successfully, but short occlusions of the iliac artery respond less well.

Antiplatelet drugs

Antiplatelet drugs are probably important in improving the patency rate after angioplasty, and aspirin 75 mg daily should be prescribed for six months after the procedure.

Complications

The associated morbidity varies from 5% to 15%. Most complications are minor, such as a haematoma at the puncture site. Thrombosis of the vessel occurs in 2-3% of patients, as does distal embolisation. Perforation of the vessel and formation of a false aneurysm are rare. The procedure has to be abandoned because of technical difficulties in between 7% and 25% of cases.

Results

The immediate success of an angioplasty can be assessed during the examination by measuring the pressure proximal and distal to the stenosis and monitoring the radiological appearances.

The aortoiliac segment—The lesion that responds best to angioplasty is a symptomatic focal stenosis of the iliac artery. Special care must be taken when the stenosis affects the orifice of another vessel (such as the internal iliac artery) as the intimal split may result in a flap, which may occlude the orifice. At the aortic bifurcation particular care must be taken to prevent damage to the other side, and to minimise this risk the "kissing" balloon technique is used. Stenosis of the internal iliac arteries that are causing impotence have been dilated with reasonable results. Iliac occlusions are on the whole not suitable for angioplasty and are best treated by operation, but the initial success rate for angioplasty of iliac stenoses is about 96%, and the five year patency has been reported to be as high as 90%.

Superficial femoral artery—Angioplasty works best for a symptomatic localised stenosis of the superficial femoral artery that is less than 2 cm long, but most patients with such lesions do well with no intervention. Longer stenoses and occlusions (of 2-15 cm) can be recanalised and dilated, however, with reasonable results. The initial success rate is significantly better for stenoses than for occlusions, but the overall initial success rate is about 85%. The long term patency also varies between stenoses and occlusions; it can be as high as 70% after five years for short segment stenoses, though it is only about 55% for occlusions. This is probably because longer stenoses and occlusions are associated with diffuse disease, making them less suitable for angioplasty.

Popliteal artery—The results in the popliteal arteries are similar to those in the superficial femoral arteries, the two year patency rate for the treatment of occlusions being between 60% and 70%. Extreme care must be taken, however, with stenoses in the distal popliteal artery because damage may result in occlusion of one or more of the crural vessels.

Angioplasty compared with operation

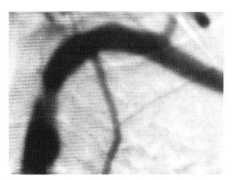

Percutaneous transluminal angioplasty is:
- Useful in localised disease
- Causes minimal morbidity
- Can be repeated if necessary

Careful consideration and discussion with the vascular surgeon are an essential part of planning treatment

It is difficult to compare angioplasty with operation. On the whole, operation is reserved for more diffuse disease and angioplasty for localised stenoses. Mortality associated with angioplasty is negligible and morbidity is low, whereas mortality after operation ranges from 1% to 5% depending on the procedure. Important advantages of angioplasty are the short inpatient stay and the low cost.

The advent of angioplasty has not, however, produced the expected savings, because more patients are now being investigated and treated. It complements rather than replaces open surgery.

Comparison of results is difficult not only because angioplasty is more suitable for patients with less severe disease but also because it fails in between 5% and 15% of patients because of technical reasons and these are usually excluded from analysis of results. Nevertheless, with favourable

Percutaneous transluminal angioplasty

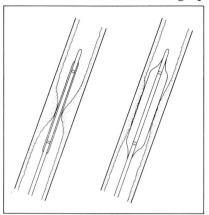

Balloon dilatation of an artery.

lesions a five year success rate of 70% for femoropopliteal dilatations and 90% for iliac dilatations (excluding technical failures) can be expected. These results compare favourably with the results for aortobifemoral and femoropopliteal grafting. It is important to recognise that the consequences of failure of angioplasty are not severe and recurrent stenoses can be redilated.

Angioplasty is now finding a role at the two extremes of the clinical range—for the patient with claudication caused by a discrete stenosis and for the patient with a critically ischaemic leg who represents a considerable operative risk. In addition, there is an increasing number of surgeons who like to perform an intraoperative iliac angioplasty before doing a femorodistal graft. Intraoperative injection of papaverine into the femoral artery (which results in relaxation of the arterioles and a reduction in femoral artery pressure if there is a more proximal stenosis) can identify those patients who require an additional procedure proximally, and angioplasty avoids retroperitoneal dissection of the iliac artery.

Angioplasty combined with other techniques

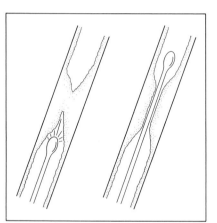

Laser used to create a channel. A balloon can then be used to dilate the track.

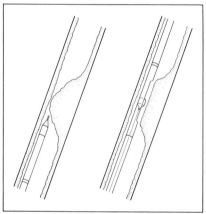

Eccentric plaque removed by atherectomy catheter.

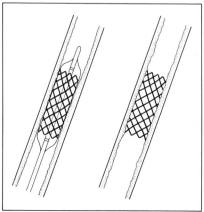

Stent inserted with a balloon catheter.

Fibrinolysis

Thrombolytic agents such as streptokinase can dissolve a recent thrombus in an artery and convert a long occlusion into a short stenosis that can be dilated by a balloon catheter. In one series the initial success rate was reported as 78% and the two year cumulative patency rate 81%, but the use of thrombolytic agents is not without risk. Complications such as diffuse bleeding and allergic reactions may be fatal. A low dose local infusion of streptokinase (5000 U/hour) reduces the systemic effect and can be useful before angioplasty in patients who are not suitable for operation. Urokinase and tissue plasminogen activator are more specific, and are not associated with allergic reactions, but they are 20 times more expensive than streptokinase. Furthermore, the current data do not show that they have any particular practical advantage.

Laser assisted angioplasty

The "hot tip" laser converts the laser energy into heat at the metal tip of the laser fibre, which burns atheroma inside the artery. Other systems use more direct laser energy and produce less damage to the vessel wall. Laser treatment was hailed as an important advance in the ablation of atheroma, but the long term results are worse than for conventional balloon procedures. The current use of lasers is limited to long occlusions in which the laser probe is used to create a channel through which balloon catheters can be advanced and balloon angioplasty done.

Atheroma cutters

High speed revolving cutters have been developed that core out atheromatous arteries; the Simpson atherectomy device was introduced in 1985 and has a side window that is positioned against the atheromatous plaque, which is then removed by the high speed cutter. The atheromatous material is stored in a special chamber in the catheter and is later removed for histopathological examination. This is ideal for localised eccentric plaques and stenoses, and a two year patency rate of 83-90% has been reported in localised iliac and femoral lesions. Other systems incorporate a rotary cutting edge at the tip of the catheter which cores out a channel through an occluded artery to facilitate the advancement of a balloon catheter.

Vascular stents

Vascular stents were developed to maintain a patent arterial lumen, but the metal mesh does not prevent reaccumulation of atheroma in the lumen of the artery and intimal hyperplasia seems to form more rapidly at the ends of the stents causing stenosis in 30-50% of cases. They are mainly used to treat recurrent stenoses or dissections, particularly in the iliac arteries, for which one year patency rates of up to 86% have been reported. The stents are not as effective in the femoral arteries, in which 57% patency after one year has been reported.

ACUTE ISCHAEMIA OF THE LEG

G A D McPherson, John H N Wolfe

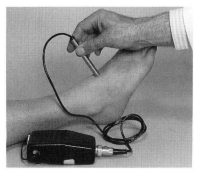
Hand held Doppler probe.

Diagnosis

Acute ischaemia of the leg is most common among elderly people, and is often diagnosed late and treated inadequately. The diagnosis should be straightforward but is often missed in its early, reversible stages. The cost to the community of a lower limb amputation is sometimes more than £25 000, and the cost to the patient may be complete disintegration of their lifestyle because they are unable to manage with their prosthetic limb.

> **Loss of pulses is the absolute criterion for acute ischaemia**

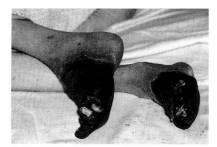
Gangrenous forefoot as a result of cold injury. Note the healthy leg and heel. Foot pulses were present.

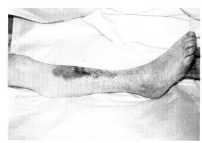
Ischaemic leg with necrotic tissue in anterior compartment and non-viable forefoot.

Symptoms and signs

The classic ischaemic limb is painful, pallid, pulseless, paraesthetic, and perished (with cold). From this the ischaemia may progress to frank gangrene with black, soggy skin within 24-48 hours. The symptoms and signs should therefore be assessed with regard to the extent, reversibility, and cause of the ischaemia.

Pain—Pain is usually severe, but in diabetic and elderly patients it may not be pronounced. The patient often gets relief of pain by hanging the leg over the edge of the bed. It is always important to find out if there is a previous history of rest pain or intermittent claudication in either leg because this suggests thrombosis rather than embolism. The pain of acute ischaemia is usually in the ischaemic muscle, which may be tender on palpation or on passive movement of the toes or foot. Pain precedes paraesthesia.

Pallor—A large femoral embolus produces a marble white leg, but more commonly an ischaemic leg is mottled. If the blue blotches do not blanch when pressed the small vessels have thrombosed and the ischaemia is probably irreversible.

Loss of pulses—In a thin patient the presence or absence of pulses is easy to establish, but it is more difficult in an obese patient, so the Doppler ultrasound probe should be used and the systolic pressure measured. Acute venous occlusion can often produce a picture that is similar to that of arterial occlusion, but with the Doppler probe it is possible to differentiate.

Paraesthesia—Sensation is not always lost, but together with absent pulses it indicates appreciable vascular occlusion that requires intervention. Diabetic patients may already have a sensory deficit which masks the change.

Paralysis—As with loss of sensation the degree of paralysis can vary, but failure of dorsiflexion of the foot is an ominous sign that suggests the need for early operation and fasciotomy.

Coldness—The patient may complain that the leg is cold, but the extent of coldness is an unreliable indicator of the level of arterial occlusion. If coldness and mottling extend to the buttock and groin, however, an aortic occlusion is likely.

Differential diagnosis

Loss of pulses is the absolute criterion for acute ischaemia. Nerve trauma, spinal disease, and cerebrovascular accidents can all simulate acute ischaemia, but these causes can usually be excluded if foot pulses are absent.

Extent

The absence of pulses is also useful in locating the occlusion. Examination of the opposite leg gives useful clues: full normal pulses suggest that embolisation is the cause, whereas absent distal pulses indicate peripheral arterial disease and the likelihood of thrombosis. Total absence

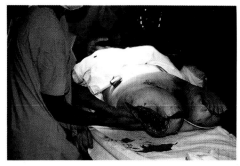

Late presentation of an aortic saddle embolus, which necessitated amputation.

Aetiology

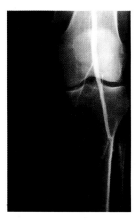

Embolus occluding the "run off" vessels from the popliteal artery.

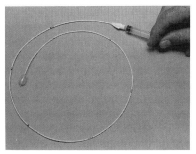

Balloon dilatation embolectomy catheter.

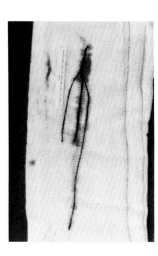

Clot removed from the popliteal and crural arteries: a successful embolectomy.

of pulses suggests a saddle embolus or thrombotic occlusion of the aorta. The diagnosis is easy in a lucid patient who presents with acute symptoms, but in an elderly, confused patient presentation may be insidious and the diagnosis easily missed.

Reversibility

The diagnosis of acute ischaemia should include an assessment not only of the level of the occlusion but also of the reversibility of the ischaemia. It is probably irreversible if there is early muscular rigidity, swelling of the foot, and blistering of the skin. Revascularisation should then be preceded by fasciotomy to ensure that the muscle is viable. Advanced skin changes such as gangrenous ulceration or crepitus are contraindications to revascularisation because this washes lethal toxins back into the circulation, and this can cause irreversible renal failure or fatal cardiac arrhythmias. If some muscles are dead they should be excised before revascularisation is attempted.

The diagnosis of acute ischaemia should include a search for the possible cause. The cause is not always clear before emergency treatment is undertaken, but the two most important causes are embolism and thrombosis of an atherosclerotic stenosis. Emergency treatment should not be undertaken without the facilities and expertise to cover any necessary procedure.

Embolism

The aetiology of embolism is changing. Before 1950, 40% of all limb emboli were caused by rheumatic heart disease; today that figure is about 8%. Nowadays cardiac emboli are commonly associated with atrial fibrillation or mural thrombus after a myocardial infarction. Rarely, the embolus arises from valve vegetations or from an atrial myxoma; the retrieved embolus should therefore always be sent for histological examination. Emboli may also arise from aneurysms, so the abdomen and popliteal fossa should be palpated carefully. Atheromatous arteries may cause distal emboli and an atheromatous abdominal aorta is a neglected source of emboli; a lateral arteriogram may show large mural thrombi.

Thrombosis

Virchow's triad of factors predisposing to thrombosis comprises changes in the wall of the vessel, changes in the constituents of the blood, and changes in the local pattern of blood flow.

Thrombosis of an atherosclerotic stenosis is the most important and most common cause of acute ischaemia. It is essential to elicit any history of claudication or rest pain, to look for the changes associated with chronic ischaemia such as loss of hair, and to examine the opposite leg for loss of pulses and the presence of bruits. Other causes of acute ischaemia include profound dehydration as a result of a massive diuresis; hyperviscosity states such as polycythaemia, thrombocythaemia, leukaemia, or myeloma; and drug induced thrombosis (in particular due to the contraceptive pill and anabolic steroids).

Trauma

Trauma is an important cause of acute ischaemia and continues to cause loss of limbs. Arterial spasm is an unacceptable diagnosis, and arteriography with a view to surgical exploration is essential if no pulses are palpable. "Arterial spasm" after a leg fracture is almost invariably caused by intimal damage and procrastination can have tragic consequences. The Doppler probe is useful but the presence of a signal does not exclude a major vascular injury.

Dissection

Arterial dissection is uncommon and difficult to diagnose. Dissections of the aorta should present with the sudden onset of searing back pain, but that is not always a predominant symptom and it is often angiography that provides the diagnosis. Once recognised the ischaemia can be reversed by a re-entry operation in which the false lumen is opened into the true lumen.

Iatrogenic dissection of a femoral, iliac, or brachial artery can occur during catheterisation. Immediate recognition and treatment should lead to complete recovery.

Management

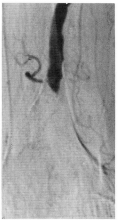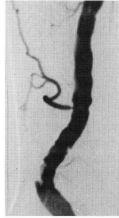

Occluded popliteal artery before (left) and after (right) treatment with intra-arterial streptokinase.

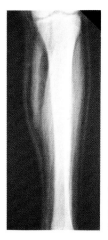

Gangrenous forefoot due to septicaemia. Surgery has no role.

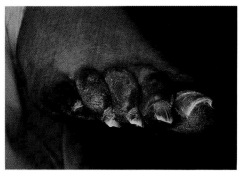

Gas gangrene in muscular planes—an absolute indication for amputation.

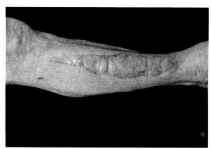

Healed anterior compartment fasciotomy—a vital adjunct to revascularisation in most patients.

Once the diagnosis has been made analgesia (15-20 mg of papaveretum intravenously) should be given. A full blood count, measurement of blood urea and potassium concentrations, and electrocardiography are essential investigations before operation. Emboli cause only a minority of cases and the surgeon should be capable of treating any eventuality.

If the ischaemia is late, delayed, and irreversible the appropriate course of action is early amputation.

Non-operative treatment

There is no doubt that an immediate embolectomy can have dramatic results even if the presentation is delayed. Patients with small vessel emboli should also be considered for operation as late complications include claudication and sometimes amputation. Non-operative treatment in the form of heparin 3000-4000 units every 24 hours or systemic streptokinase have been recommended. The success rate is low, however, at around 30%, and there is a high incidence of sensitivity reactions and bleeding. Urokinase overcomes the sensitivity reactions but not the bleeding problems and is extremely expensive.

Low dose intra-arterial infusion of streptokinase (5000 U/hour) is of value if the tip of the catheter is placed at the occlusion, and the results of clot lysis with tissue plasminogen activator have also been encouraging, though this is also expensive. If there is time for lysis this has the considerable advantage of delineating the sort of localised stenosis that requires limited operation and, occasionally, operation can be avoided completely.

Percutaneous aspiration of clot is another recent advance. The technique requires further assessment, though it may be of particular use in treating the catheter induced thrombosis that can occur during angiography and angioplasty.

Operation should be considered in all patients with acute ischaemia if it is uncertain whether the leg will survive another 6-12 hours (the muscles are tender and immobile and there is extensive paraesthesia). Acute on chronic ischaemia is often less of an emergency, and lysis of the clot should show the focal lesion that can then be dealt with either by balloon dilatation or by limited operation. Ischaemia as a result of occlusion of a femoropopliteal graft is usually best treated by clot lysis so that the offending stenosis and "run off" arteries can be seen, thus simplifying the subsequent reconstruction.

Operative treatment of acute ischaemia

As a rule angiography should be done before operation, but if this is not possible it should be done during the operation. Often patients are in advanced cardiac failure, and appropriate treatment should be given. General anaesthesia is preferable to local anaesthesia because operative approaches to the infrainguinal vessels are easier and access to vessels above the groin is then possible. Local anaesthesia is sometimes necessary, however, for elderly ill patients with advanced cardiac disease and should comprise local infiltration with lignocaine 0·5% and intravenous diazepam (Diazemuls) for sedation. An anaesthetist should be present at the operation.

Femoral embolectomy—The embolus can sometimes be removed with forceps and gentle digital manipulation, but a Fogarty balloon catheter should be used to unblock distal vessels. This procedure is often successful but must be done with great care because overinflation of the balloon can damage or even rupture the arterial wall, as can vigorous pulling on the catheter. After removal of the catheter it is always advisable to irrigate the vessels with heparinised saline—some catheters have an irrigation port that opens beyond the balloon so that this can be done easily. If it is impossible to pass the catheter angiography should be used to find out the nature of the block, which is usually atherosclerotic. An angiogram should also be done when the catheter is passed because if there is no backflow on removal of the catheter, or if the catheter does not pass through into the crural vessels, it is of help in deciding whether to explore the popliteal artery and proceed to arterial reconstruction. Increasingly, distal clots are being treated by intraoperative intra-arterial streptokinase (100 000 units); this is a daunting technique, but seems to be safe and effective.

Embolectomy with fasciotomy—If the presentation is delayed the embolus

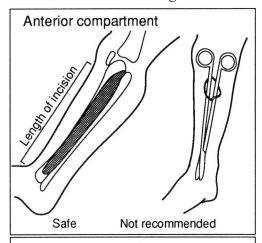

Anterior compartment

Length of incision

Safe   Not recommended

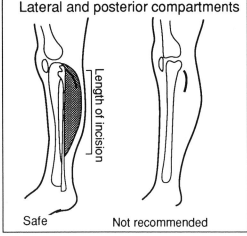

Lateral and posterior compartments

Length of incision

Safe   Not recommended

Fasciotomy.

is likely to be more adherent and may require multiple arteriotomies. In one report of patients in whom presentation was delayed up to 63 days successful embolectomies were done in two thirds. In all such patients fasciotomy should be considered. Red, glossy skin with tender, swollen muscles and symptoms that have lasted for 24 hours indicate that the muscles are under tension and at risk of necrosis. Fasciotomy in which the anterior, lateral, and posterior compartments are split is simple to do and too often omitted. The skin incision should be full length to ensure that the fascia is adequately incised.

Postoperatively the aim should be to save the patient's life. A quarter of all patients who undergo femoral embolectomy die in hospital, and a further 16% require an amputation. Cardiac failure must be treated and the patient should have physiotherapy to the chest and the limb. The foot should rest on a sheepskin and be protected by a cradle. Roughly half of the postoperative deaths are caused by thromboembolic complications, so the patient should receive anticoagulant drugs from the time of operation initially with heparin 20 000-40 000 units/24 hours for one week, followed by warfarin for three months.

Thrombectomy and reconstruction for atherosclerotic stenoses

There are two alternative treatments for acute thrombosis of an atherosclerotic stenosis: thrombectomy followed by early planned reconstructive surgery or thrombectomy with immediate reconstruction. Angiography provides the essential aid in deciding which to choose.

If the common femoral artery is severely atheromatous a local femoral endarterectomy or vein patch may be necessary. If the superficial femoral artery is occluded but the profunda is widely patent with good backflow the limb will remain viable with thrombectomy alone. If the inflow to the femoral artery is reduced a femorofemoral crossover graft may be better tolerated than operation on the aortoiliac segment. A femoropopliteal bypass graft is indicated if the outflow is poor. When the popliteal artery is blocked a femorodistal graft to one of the crural vessels is usually possible even if the angiogram does not identify a patent vessel.

The success rate of reconstructive operations largely depends on adequate angiography. Peroperative angiography provides good visualisation of distal vessels, but preoperative arteriography is necessary for any assessment of the aortoiliac segment.

Outcome

> **A quarter of all patients die in hospital after femoral embolectomy**

The outcome of acute ischaemia depends on two factors—the general state of the patient and the duration of the ischaemia. If the patient is elderly with advanced cardiac disease the outcome is poor, and it is this group of patients that accounts for the overall mortality of 25%. The primary object of treatment should therefore be to save the patient by treating cardiac failure and improving the respiratory function. The duration of ischaemia is critical after 24 hours. If the patient is treated within 24 hours the amputation rate is only 9%, but after that it rises to 23%.

CRITICAL LEG ISCHAEMIA: AMPUTATION OR RECONSTRUCTION

N J W Cheshire, John H N Wolfe

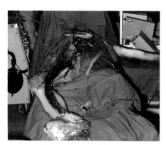

Reconstruction of aortoiliac segment and femoroperoneal graft. Such an extensive operation is now sometimes indicated.

The number of major amputations done each year for vascular insufficiency is not precisely known but is probably about 10 000. This suggests that between 20% and 40% of all critically ischaemic legs are amputated eventually.

Society's attitudes to amputation have changed little since mediaeval times, and patients' responses to loss of a limb remain nearly as dramatic as to the announcement of terminal illness. Recent advances in vascular surgery have led us to reappraise the optimal management of critical leg ischaemia and in this article we consider the roles of amputation and revascularisation.

Surgical options

Most, though not all, patients with critically ischaemic legs require successful arterial reconstruction if major amputation is to be avoided. Management depends on the site of the stenosis or occlusion. Certain options are preferable at particular sites, but effective reconstruction often requires simultaneous or serial application of several techniques.

30% Balloon dilatation
Aortobifemoral graft
Axillobifemoral graft
Unilateral: femorofemoral
crossover graft
Unilateral: iliofemoral graft

40% Balloon dilatation, with or
without atherectomy
Femoropopliteal bypass graft
Profundaplasty

30% Femorocrural /pedal
bypass graft
Popliteal-crural /pedal
bypass graft

Alternatives to amputation for ischaemia of the lower limb.

Aortoiliac reconstruction

Aortoiliac disease readily responds to reconstruction. Techniques of percutaneous angioplasty are effective for patients with short occlusions or stenoses and can be repeated if they restenose. Arterial grafts in this region have high patency rates (95% at five years) with a low incidence of reoperation. In a particularly frail patient insertion of an extra-anatomic axillofemoral graft is less traumatic but has a lower patency rate (70% at one year). Revascularisation for aortoiliac disease is therefore justified, and few surgeons would deny reconstruction to a patient with occlusion in this arterial segment.

Femoropopliteal reconstruction

Percutaneous techniques are not as effective for revascularisation of the femoropopliteal segment as they are for the aortoiliac segment. Although balloon dilatation has a role in the management of localised stenoses of the superficial femoral artery, an isolated lesion of this type rarely produces critical ischaemia. Several people are working on the development of percutaneous atherectomy, but reported results vary. Most patients therefore undergo femoropopliteal bypass.

Patency rates at three years range from 80% for autologous vein bypass to the proximal popliteal artery to 55% for prosthetic bypass to the distal popliteal artery. These figures can be maintained over many years if there is a surveillance programme to detect stenoses within the graft. Such favourable results mean that most patients with femoropopliteal disease should be offered revascularisation if the viability of the limb is threatened.

Critical leg ischaemia: amputation or reconstruction

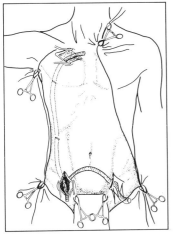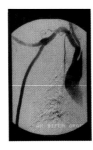

Axillobifemoral graft. Operative diagram (left) and postoperative angiogram (right) showing graft originating from proximal axillary artery.

When a viable limb does not confer any advantage because the patient is already totally dependent, however, the risk:benefit ratio is altered and primary amputation may be appropriate.

Femorocrural reconstruction

When occlusive vascular disease extends beyond the popliteal artery into the three crural vessels (the peroneal artery and the anterior and posterior tibial arteries) percutaneous techniques are of no value in primary revascularisation. We therefore insert a femorocrural bypass graft or—rarely—deem the disease unreconstructable and carry out a primary amputation. Grafts at this level often fail, and the patient's morale is sapped by a series of revisions followed by major amputation. It is therefore in patients with distal disease that we need to look closely at comparisons in outcome between modern reconstruction and amputation if we are to provide the patient with the best chance of returning to normal life.

Femorocrural reconstruction compared with amputation

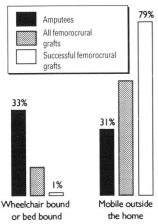

- Amputees
- All femorocrural grafts
- Successful femorocrural grafts

79%

33%

31%

1%

Wheelchair bound or bed bound

Mobile outside the home

Mobility after three years in patients with femorocrural grafts compared with amputees.

Autologous vein can be harvested from the long saphenous in either leg, the short saphenous vein, or an arm vein. If a thorough search is made it is usually possible to construct a long femorocrural graft with vein, but on some occasions (particularly if there has been more than one previous operation) an adequate amount of vein cannot be found. The patency rates for vein grafts may be as high as 70% at one year and 60% at three years, but if prosthetic material is used for these long grafts the results are not nearly as good. The use of a venous collar seems to improve the patency rates of femorocrural prosthetic grafts, however, and patency rates 20% worse than those for vein grafts are now being achieved.

Mortality

Early reports of long term survival in patients who presented with critical leg ischaemia suggested a five year mortality of 40%-100% regardless of management. More recently, however, improved survival rates have been reported; up to 80% of patients may be expected to survive for three years and we must consider this when recommending treatment. Mortality within 30 days after reconstruction compares favourably with that after amputation (1% compared with 10% in our current practice), and this improvement is presumably a consequence of the aggressive management of vascular disease in other areas of the body, notably the coronary circulation.

Femorocrural reconstruction can therefore be undertaken safely in patients with critical leg ischaemia. This operation has implications for a large proportion of patients, most of whom will survive for some years after their operations.

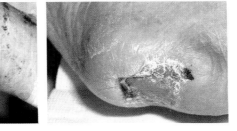

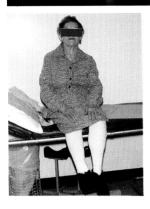

Necrotic ulcer of the heel (top left): a femoroperoneal vein graft and removal of part of the calcaneus followed by skin grafting (top right) resulted in full rehabilitation (left).

Mobility

Successful reconstruction has been associated with excellent mobility; almost four fifths of patients could walk independently outside their homes. Conversely, mobility after amputation was poor with less than a third of patients walking independently outside their homes, and over a third being confined to a wheelchair or bed. Poor mobility after amputation has now been reported from several centres at which geriatric patients are treated, and these results have important implications for everybody concerned with the management of leg ischaemia.

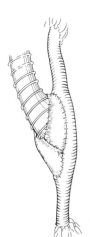

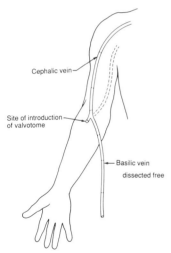

Diagram (left) and radiograph (below) showing vein collar used to improve patency of distal prosthetic graft.

Conclusion

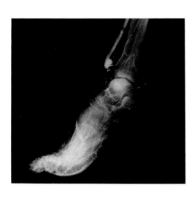

Even if the veins in the forearm are thrombosed, extensive lengths of vein can be obtained from the upper arm.

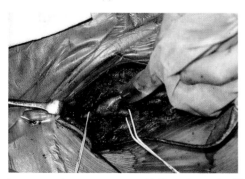

Intraoperative assessment with Doppler probe. This cheap instrument can be inserted in a sterile glove to scan the graft for abnormalities in flow at the end of the operation.

Limb salvage and graft patency

At follow up after three years 72% of vein grafts and 51% of prosthetic grafts were still viable (97% of irreversible graft failures resulted in major amputations). Further operations to maintain the patency of the grafts was required in 15% of patients during subsequent years and they avoided amputation. These reinterventions depend on a graft surveillance programme in which stenoses in the grafts are identified by treadmill Doppler studies, duplex scanning, or intravenous digital subtraction angiography. We rely on duplex scanning, which must be carried out twice within the first six months of operation to be of any value as almost all graft stenoses develop within the first year.

These patency figures were achieved in a relatively unselected group of patients in whom scrupulous attention was paid to graft follow up, correction of intragraft stenoses, correction of polycythaemia, and appropriate anticoagulation. Many of the patients stopped smoking because the dire consequences were so obvious, and stopping smoking is now of confirmed benefit.

Costs

Analysis of the cost of each option is now an integral part of health care. Assessment of the cost of vascular reconstruction must accommodate the primary operation and all subsequent procedures (including the cost of secondary amputation when necessary). The primary reconstruction is only one third of the cost of amputation, but when subsequent operations (including some major amputations) are also considered, the cost of grafting veins to distal crural vessels more than doubles. Using these grafts routinely is nevertheless cheaper than doing primary amputations. Even when the higher rates of failure and reintervention that are associated with prosthetic grafting are included, the overall cost of reconstruction is less than that of amputation.

We advise revascularisation for almost all patients who present with aortoiliac or femoropopliteal occlusive disease and limb threatening ischaemia. In addition, we now also suggest reconstruction to the distal crural vessels; this affects about one third of patients. Femorocrural bypass grafts can be inserted with a low operative mortality, and they result in vastly improved mobility compared with amputation. In addition, these grafts give acceptable rates of limb salvage and graft patency at medium term follow up (even when prosthetic grafts are used) and can be done for less than the cost of amputation.

Given most patients' undoubted objection to amputation we believe that revascularisation should be offered to almost all those with limb threatening ischaemia unless the patient's quality of life will not be improved by saving the leg.

REHABILITATION OF THE AMPUTEE

S J D Chadwick, John H N Wolfe

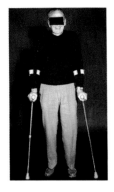

A successful above knee amputation. The patient was walking on crutches within 10 days of operation. He had run eight miles a day until acute thrombosis of a popliteal aneurysm produced irreversible ischaemia.

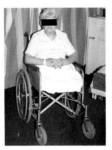

A bilateral above knee amputee who was confined to a wheelchair but remained motivated and relatively independent.

Most lower limb amputations are now done because of vascular insufficiency. In 1987, 4985 new lower limb amputees were referred to the disablement service centres (previously known as artificial limb and appliance centres) in England. Two thirds of these amputations were done for peripheral vascular disease and more than a fifth for the complications of diabetes mellitus. About 80% of the patients were over 60 years old at the time of amputation. The problems to be faced after amputation, therefore, are not only those of achieving independent mobility, but also of managing illnesses associated with advancing years and returning to the community.

There are three important aims:
- To produce a soundly healed stump and a patient who can walk. The level of amputation is therefore crucial: above the knee amputations heal readily but many patients who have them never master walking on a prosthesis. The converse is true of below knee amputations
- Early rehabilitation with a prosthesis
- Cost effectiveness.

These may be achieved with a hospital based rehabilitation team that liaises closely with the disablement service centre, the general practitioner, and the community services.

Process of rehabilitation

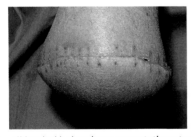

A well healed below knee amputation stump. The muscularity of the leg has not been adequately accounted for, resulting in a bulky stump that is difficult to fit with a prosthesis.

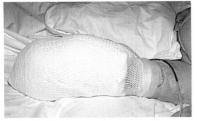

The ideal initial stump dressing using cotton wool, Netelast, and no tape. A poor crepe can occlude venous drainage and produce stump oedema.

Before the stump has healed

Early referral of a patient with critical ischaemia of the lower limb to a specialist vascular surgeon is essential so that either salvage of the limb by reconstructive surgery or interventional radiology may be attempted, and (if these are not possible) sufficient time will be available to prepare the patient for amputation.

Compression bandaging should not be used on the stump during the early postoperative period while it is healing. The patient should be mobilised by using the pneumatic post amputation mobility aid (PPAM aid) under the supervision of an experienced physiotherapist. Initially, he or she should use parallel bars for support, and then graduate to elbow crutches. The patient will then be referred to the local disablement service centre to be assessed and measured for a prosthesis, unless it is thought that walking is unlikely, in which case a wheelchair will be provided.

Mobilisation

Those who can walk are taught how to cope. The Department of Health has produced a booklet called *Your next step forward*. It is an introduction to the disablement service centre, and gives information about the services available and how to care for the stump and the artificial limb. Good communication between the hospital, the disablement service centre, and the general practitioner is essential.

When the stump is soundly healed the patient will receive his or her first artificial limb—usually a definitive prosthesis with a temporary socket. Occasionally a temporary or pylon limb may be used—for example, for patients who are frail and require the lightest possible prosthesis, or for those in whom there is doubt about whether they will use a prosthesis. During this rehabilitation phase patients are shown how to care for the

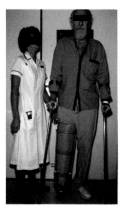

Once the suture line has healed a pneumatic post-amputation mobility aid is excellent for early walking.

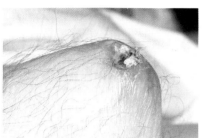

Poor above knee stump with retraction of muscle and erosion of bone through the skin.

The amputated limb

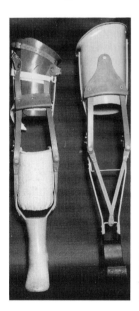

A below knee (left) and above knee (right) rocker pylon that can be used while the final prosthesis is being built.

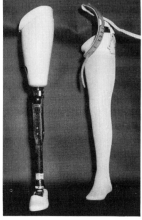

An Endolite above knee prosthesis with suction socket at the fitting stage and with the external cover and rigid pelvic strap.

stump, put on the artificial limb, and dress. The length of time they spend standing is increased, and they learn to walk—at first on the flat and later on sloping and uneven surfaces—and to pick up objects from the floor and to climb stairs. They are taught how to pick themselves up after falling over. Close supervision is therefore essential. The occupational therapist and social worker will by this time have visited their homes and assessed what structural changes will be required or if reaccommodation is necessary.

Progress is discussed at regular meetings of the rehabilitation team. Before discharge from hospital not only must the patients be independently mobile, but also the place to which they are going (their own home, or the home of family or friends) must be prepared. The community services—provided by the district nurse, the home help, and "meals on wheels"—should be arranged before discharge, when close liaison with the general practitioner is vital so that continuity of care and support are maintained. The general practitioners should be in a position to smooth over any of the initial fears that the families may have about accepting amputees back into the home.

After discharge from hospital

Amputation causes a considerable change in body symmetry, which will affect both the posture and the body image. Most patients seem to adjust well to life with an artificial limb, though there are three topics on which medical advice and help may be sought: the amputated limb, general health, and social activities.

The stump

The stump is a vulnerable area that requires great care and attention.

General care—An amputee will have been taught how to care for the stump (including simple hygienic measures) in the hospital and at the disablement service centre. The stump usually takes a few months to mature, so that in the early period after discharge from hospital it should be examined regularly for oedema and infection. Swelling should be controlled by stump compression socks. Bandages should be applied to the stump only by those skilled in the technique. Infection should be treated with rest and antibiotics. Stump socks are provided, and the choice of material is decided by the fit of the limb to avoid chaffing and not by the patient's preference. Problems with the weight bearing areas of the stump and the interface of the prosthesis will arise as the stump shrinks and the socket becomes loose. An amputee should be advised to wear more than one stump sock, and an appointment should be made at the disablement service centre for adjustment of the socket.

Stump pain—Neuromas may cause pains varying from dull aches to electric shocks. Transcutaneous nerve stimulation may relieve the symptoms, but excision may be required. Pain may also be caused by osteomyelitis, the growth of a bony spur, or ischaemia. Radiographs will confirm the diagnosis of the first two, but if ischaemia is suspected an urgent appointment with the surgeon is indicated. Pain from the lumbar spine may result from tilting of the pelvis because the artificial limb is too short or because the gait is unsatisfactory. In such cases the amputee should be referred to the disablement service centre for treatment.

Phantom limb pain

Most patients experience phantom pains, which can be depressing. Reassurance, carbamazepine, transcutaneous nerve stimulation, tapping the stump, and acupuncture have all been tried with varying degrees of success, but the symptoms may become blunted with time. Carbamazepine is usually the first line of treatment and is often effective.

Discomfort from the prosthesis

Discomfort from the buckles and straps of the prosthesis, and generalised aches and pains associated with the use of the prosthesis are common. An above the knee amputee may be given a prosthesis that has a waistband and shoulder strap, which may cause pain from chaffing and pressure. One simple cure is to pad out the straps. Alternatively, the doctor at the disablement service centre may prescribe a suction socket, thereby

Rehabilitation of the amputee

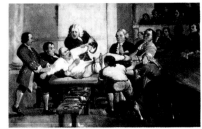

"The horror of surgery must be minimised by careful counselling." An amputation performed without anaesthesia at St Thomas's Hospital in the nineteenth century.

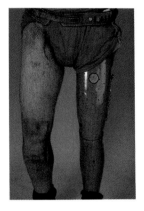

Buckles and strap from an above knee prosthesis may rub on the operation scar of the contralateral arterial reconstruction.

Social activities

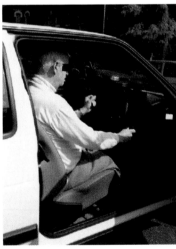

Bilateral above knee amputation does not preclude driving and independence.

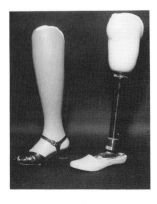

An Endolite supracondyle patella bearing prosthesis in the fitting stage (right) and with external cover (left).

removing the necessity for straps. As most of the patients are elderly, however, their stumps and general health usually preclude the use of suction sockets. Where possible analgesics (which may cause constipation) should be avoided. Instead regular physiotherapy or osteopathy should be prescribed.

Psychological effects

Loss of a limb has been described in the same emotional terms as a bereavement; these feelings are intensified by phantom limb sensations, and are more pronounced in elderly people. If the explanation of why the limb was amputated has not been accepted by the patient he or she may blame the medical staff for the disability. This is not always a hostile reaction and may be expressed as a demand for extra attention. Psychiatric help may occasionally be needed.

Care of the artificial limb

This is entirely within the province of the disablement service centres, which offer a service throughout the United Kingdom even when the amputee is away from home. If damage or breakdown occurs the patient may telephone the local disablement service centre to arrange an appointment.

General health of the amputee

Although the long term prognosis of patients who have had amputations for peripheral vascular disease is poor, it is essential to maintain their dignity and health. Problems of aging (such as prostatic hypertrophy causing nocturia) need prompt treatment. Attention must be paid to controlling conditions that may have a deleterious effect on the stump, the remaining limbs, and mobility—for example, diabetes mellitus, cardiorespiratory disease, and arthritis. Clearly it is imperative that every effort is made to prevent irreversible ischaemia in the remaining leg. If a new condition is diagnosed the disablement service centre should be informed.

Work

Amputees who wish to return to work should be encouraged to do so. If they are unable to take up their original employment the disablement resettlement officer should be contacted.

Driving

Amputees must inform the Driver and Vehicle Licensing Centre (DVLC) and their insurance company about their disability, but the amputation will not debar them from driving as the car can be modified. The licensing centre stipulates that automatic transmission is preferable. For a bilateral amputee hand controls are required. The amputee should be advised to contact the British School of Motoring or a local agency recommended by the disablement service centre for a trial assessment and should join the Disabled Drivers' Association, members of which will give practical advice.

Public transport

Getting on or off buses and escalators should initially be supervised by an occupational therapist. Many elderly amputees never manage without help.

Shoes

The soles and heels of any new shoes require close scrutiny. When the heel is flat on the ground the sole must be as well otherwise the gait may be altered. The disablement service centre can adjust the height of a prosthesis if the patient wishes to use heels of different heights, and there is an adjustable heel device that can be fitted to many limbs so that the patients may adjust the height of the heel themselves.

Leisure activities

After spending some time in hospital most patients gain weight. Amputees should therefore be encouraged to take up some form of physical exercise.

Holidays

Amputees should be advised to take crutches when they travel away from home in case of mechanical failure of the limb. If spending their holidays within the United Kingdom they should obtain the telephone number of the nearest disablement service centre, which will always carry out emergency repairs; if going abroad they should make inquiries about reciprocal repair arrangements.

Conclusion

Useful addresses:

The Royal Association For Disability and Rehabilitation (RADAR), 25 Mortimer Street, London W1 8AB, tel: 071-637 5400

British Limbless Ex-Servicemen's Association (BLESMA), 185-187 High Road, Frankland Moore House, Chadwell Heath, Essex RM6 6NA, tel: 081-590-1124

National Association for Limbless Disabled (NALD), 31, The Mall, Ealing, London, W5 2PX, tel: 081-579-1758/9

Useful publications:

If Only I'd Known That a Year Ago. . . . . published by RADAR. This booklet reviews what is available to disabled people, their families, and friends and includes the addresses of many useful organisations and associations

Driving after amputation and *How to get behind the wheel* are both published by Forum of Driving Assessment Centres, c/o Banstead Mobility Centre, Damson Way, Orchard Hill, Queen Mary's Avenue, Carshalton, Surrey SM5 4NR, tel: 081-770-1151

The artificial limb and appliance centres were criticised in a report published in 1987 to the Department of Health by a committee chaired by Lord McColl. The committee suggested that the service could be improved by raising the technical standards of amputation; by setting up specialist multidisciplinary hospital teams that would work in close cooperation with the medical staff at the centres and take an active part in rehabilitation; by giving more responsibility to prosthetists and encouraging them to be responsible for continuing care; and, finally, by restructuring of management. Some changes have already been implemented—such as the integration of the service into health regions with integrated budgets. Prosthetists may now tender for provision and service contracts, thus allowing them to become independent of the major suppliers of artificial limbs.

The demands of amputees on the medical and associated services will vary according to their independence. Some will need little medical help; a new elderly amputee, however, will require extensive support and supervision if he or she is to be discharged from an acute hospital and return to the community. After discharge from hospital the general practitioner will not only look after the immediate physical requirements of the amputee but also coordinate the community support, the hospital services, and the services of the disablement service centre.

We thank Mr Kiril Gray and Mr Ray Holland (BLESMA) for their help, and Dr Linda Marks of the DSA limb fitting centre, Stanmore, for her criticisms and comments. We are grateful to the Royal College of Surgeons of England for permission to reproduce the picture of the amputation in the eighteenth century.

THE DIABETIC FOOT

R S Elkeles, John H N Wolfe

Infection

Ischaemia ——— Neuropathy

More hospital beds in Britain are occupied by diabetic patients with disorders of their feet than by patients with all the other complications of diabetes combined (despite the fact that diabetes is also one of the most common causes of both renal failure and blindness). The two main features are neuropathy and ischaemia, both of which predispose to infection and lead to necrosis of the tissue. They are often present together.

The management of the diabetic foot requires the combined skills of a number of people: general practitioner, diabetic physician, vascular surgeon, orthopaedic surgeon, chiropodist, nurse, microbiologist, physiotherapist, surgical footwear specialist, and limb fitter. Every effort should be made to make sure that this team works together.

The neuropathic foot

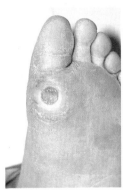

The commonest site of a neuropathic ulcer. The toes do not look ischaemic.

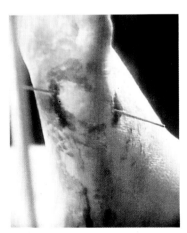

Extensive destruction of tissue beneath small lesions, with needle running along track between plantar and dorsal ulcers.

The most common serious complication of diabetic peripheral neuropathy that affects the foot is the neuropathic ulcer. Loss of sensation results in failure to perceive damage caused by mechanical trauma—for example, friction from badly fitting shoes, penetration of sharp objects on the floor, or heat from radiators or fires. Neuropathy also stops the intrinsic muscles of the foot from opposing the long muscles, which leads to the "claw toe" deformity and transfers weight bearing from the toes to the heads of the metatarsals. The condition is exacerbated by the microcirculatory abnormalities in the skin that may predispose to ulceration. Pressure on the plantar skin is increased and callus builds up under the heads of one or more metatarsals. Fluid collects underneath the callus and infection may then supervene, leading to abscess formation and ulceration. It is important to appreciate that—unlike with most other ulcers—the initial problem is the formation of a cavity deep to the epithelium, which is followed by ulceration. The initial event is the formation of a plaque of hard keratin, and the tissues break down underneath this. A cavity filled with plasma and blood then develops, enlarges, and eventually ruptures on to the skin surface. The ulcerated opening is therefore small compared with the large cavity beneath. This ulcer may remain uninfected for a prolonged period, but if the opening to the cavity becomes occluded with keratin and inspissated discharge, then overt infection may develop rapidly and progress at an alarming rate to affect the underlying tendon and bone.

The problem is further complicated by alteration to both the structure and function of proteins in diabetic patients. Hyperglycaemia produces non-enzymatic glycosylation of collagen and keratin. These tissues then become more rigid and inflexible, and resistant to enzymatic digestion by collagenase. Keratin is not readily removed from the superficial layers of the sole of the foot and hyperkeratosis develops. The abnormal collagen is highly inflexible so that shear stresses on the pressure points lead to tissue breakdown and eventual ulceration.

Healing of this ulceration is also impaired in diabetic patients. Their raised tissue glucose concentrations reduce the activity of leucocytes and macrophages, which fail to produce enough fibroblasts to synthesise the collagen.

On clinical examination the diabetic neuropathic foot is warm, pink, and dry with easily palpable pulses. Tendon reflexes are impaired and sensation to vibration, pinprick, and light touch is reduced.

Management

Infection—Infections are almost invariably associated with a mixture of Gram positive, Gram negative, enteric, and anaerobic organisms. As about 70% of infected ulcers contain anaerobic organisms systemic treatment is essential. Swabs should be taken from the ulcer before antimicrobial agents are prescribed. If there is spreading cellulitis blood should be cultured. A patient with superficial ulceration can be treated with systemic antibiotics, cleansing of the ulcer, and application of non-adhesive dressings as an outpatient, but the importance of restricting activity until the inflammation has settled must be emphasised. More serious infections require admission to hospital for bed rest and intravenous antibiotics. A combination of benzylpenicillin, ampicillin, and metronidazole is usually given until results of the cultures are available, when a more appropriate choice can be made.

Removal of necrotic tissue—A grossly infected neuropathic foot with osteomyelitis of the metatarsals can usually be saved, so any foot that is not ischaemic should be managed conservatively. Initially the infection should be drained and irrigated, frankly necrotic tissue should be removed, antibiotics given, and the patient confined to bed. An attempt to remove all the infected and inflamed tissue at this stage may result in unnecessary extensive destruction of tendons in the foot, and the resulting deformity may make it difficult to prevent further damage to pressure points. Once the infection has been drained and controlled it is possible to assess the extent of damage to the tissues, and the cavity can be carefully pared back to healthy tissue. Every effort should be made to preserve viable skin to close the defect.

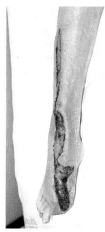

Extensive infection tracking up the anterior compartment of the leg. After debridement and skin grafting the leg was saved.

<table>
<tr><td colspan="2">

Care of the feet

1 Do not walk barefoot

2 Wash your feet daily with soap and warm but not hot water. Dry well with a soft towel, especially between toes

3 Check your feet daily for skin cracks or blisters. If you cannot see the soles use a mirror or ask someone else to look

4 Check that shoes are not too tight or too loose. Take special care with new shoes. Wear new shoes for only short periods initially. Check inside new shoes for any loose object or roughness on the insole before putting them on

5 If your sight is poor or if you find it difficult to reach your toenails get the chiropodist to cut them

6 Do not sit close to fires or radiators and do not have a hot water bottle in bed

7 Change socks or stockings daily. These should be loose fitting, and in cold weather wear woollen ones

8 Do not use corn plasters or paints. Visit the chiropodist regularly

</td></tr>
</table>

Control of diabetes—It is likely that control of the diabetes helps to reduce the spread of infection, but control of diabetes is itself made more difficult by infection. A patient who has been treated with diet only or with diet and tablets will usually require insulin during these periods of infection, given either by intravenous infusion or multiple subcutaneous injections.

Redistribution of weight—Neuropathic ulcers often take weeks or months to heal, and the only way to ensure healing is to remove weight bearing and friction from the ulcerated areas. In practice this is difficult. Bed rest is the surest way in the short term, but in the long term it can be extremely trying for the patient and (in these days of extreme shortage of beds) difficult and costly. An alternative when the infection has been treated and the ulcer cleaned is to apply a below knee plaster with forward projection of the cast to the level of the mid-shaft of the proximal phalanges of the toes. This permits the ulcer to be inspected and dressed.

Because of the sensory neuropathy, extra foam padding must be put under the plaster. By this technique patients can be mobile while healing is taking place. Other methods include wearing moulded insoles or a semirigid boot of synthetic material with a piece cut out over the ulcer.

Once the ulceration has healed the redistribution of stress must be maintained by moulded insoles to prevent recurrent ulceration.

Radiograph showing bony destruction, particularly of the fifth metatarsal, and gas in the tissues as a result of ulceration.

Other complications

Painful diabetic neuropathy—Though most diabetic peripheral neuropathy is painless, some patients have severe pain in the legs and feet; treatment of this is difficult and unsatisfactory. Optimal control of the diabetes is the first essential, together with simple analgesics and combinations of phenothiazines and antidepressants. Achievement of adequate sleep with night sedation is important. A new class of drugs, the aldose reductase inhibitors (which reduce accumulation of sorbitol in nerves affected by diabetes), is currently being evaluated in clinical trials.

Charcot's joints—Neurogenic arthropathy is a rare complication of diabetes that results in destruction of bones and joints leading to severe deformity of the foot.

The ischaemic foot

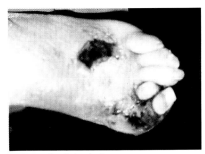

Ischaemic diabetic foot.

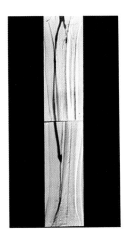

Angiogram of vein bypass graft from popliteal to posterior tibial artery. The popliteal pulse was present but the foot was ischaemic.

Ischaemia in a diabetic foot is caused by atherosclerosis, which is more common among diabetic patients than non-diabetic patients. The occlusive arterial disease occurs in younger patients and in a more severe form than in non-diabetic patients and it is more often bilateral. Furthermore, diabetic patients tend to have hypercoagulable blood. The symptoms are intermittent claudication and—later—rest pain, which may be followed by ulceration and gangrene. In contrast to the neuropathic foot, the ischaemic foot is cool with shiny red atrophic skin and absent peripheral pulses.

Management

Investigations—Doppler ultrasound pressure wave measurements of the ankle to arm systolic blood pressure ratio provide a simple non-invasive way of confirming the presence of peripheral vascular disease. Unfortunately the calcification that develops in these diabetic patients' vessels may make the vessels incompressible under the sphygmomanometer cuff and give spuriously normal readings. Arteriography is required if reconstructive surgery is to be considered. The presence of a palpable popliteal pulse is no longer a contraindication to arteriography, and if the femoral pulse is normal the radiologist should concentrate on the lower leg arteries, including those in the foot.

Medical management—Claudication is often mild and intermittent and may go on for years without progressing, and medical management has an important part to play. The patient must stop smoking, and control of the diabetes should be optimal. Infection should be treated early, and β blockers should be avoided if possible. Suitable protective footwear should be worn and chiropody should be arranged. If the patient is obese, weight reduction should be encouraged until the weight is close to the ideal (which will also help improve control of the diabetes).

Surgical management—The previous pessimism about treating distal arterial occlusions by operation has been mitigated by improved techniques. Worthwhile results can now be expected if a vein graft can be anastomosed to a single patent vessel at the level of the ankle. A routine arteriogram may fail to opacify these vessels, but new arteriographic and Doppler techniques will show vessels that can be used for reconstruction. The "in situ" vein technique has helped, but arm veins may also be used and short bypasses from the popliteal artery to the ankle are also worth while.

Conclusion

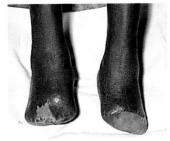

Bilateral leg revascularisation resulting in successful transmetatarsal amputations.

The physician must be constantly alert to the development of peripheral neuropathy or vascular disease in diabetic patients. Examination of the feet should be part of every review in the diabetic clinic. Once a problem has arisen the patient should be instructed in the care of his or her feet. The patient should wear broad fitting shoes with low broad heels and soft uppers. There should be no pressure points. Printed instructions should be given to these patients.

We thank Upjohn for permission to reproduce the photograph depicting extensive destruction of tissue beneath small lesions, and the radiograph of the foot.

TREATING AORTIC ANEURYSMS

P R Taylor, John H N Wolfe

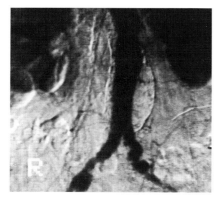

Digital subtraction angiogram showing contrast in the aorta and diseased iliac arteries. The thrombus in the aneurysmal sac is to the right of the aortic lumen.

Rupture of an abdominal aortic aneurysm remains one of the most dangerous events in vascular surgery, the mortality being close to 100% if the condition is not treated. The diagnosis may, however, be difficult as many other life threatening conditions produce a similar clinical picture. Any delay in operating on these patients has a serious adverse effect on their outcome; many die before they reach the operating theatre, so the mortality in the community remains over 90%. Furthermore, the perioperative mortality has remained constant at 30-50% despite advances in anaesthetic and surgical techniques during the past two decades.

In contrast, mortality after elective repair of an aneurysm that has not ruptured is usually between 2% and 5%. Even operations on selected patients over the age of 80 have a mortality of only about 10%. The most important way of improving the poor prognosis of patients with ruptured abdominal aortic aneurysms is to diagnose the aneurysm before it ruptures. Careful assessment by surgeons and cardiologists can then be made before operation is contemplated.

Incidence

Differential diagnoses for ruptured abdominal aortic aneurysm

- Myocardial ischaemia
- Perforated ulcer
- Acute cholecystitis
- Acute pancreatitis
- Renal or ureteric colic
- Bowel obstruction

The incidence of abdominal aortic aneurysm is increasing in the United Kingdom; it is more common among men than women, the ratio being about 5:1. Although the natural course is unknown, aneurysms expand at a rate of about 0·5 cm a year, which increases as the aneurysm enlarges. The risk of rupture increases proportionately with the diameter, but even aneurysms <4 cm have a slight risk of rupture. Less than half the patients with symptomatic aneurysms will survive a year, and asymptomatic aneurysms also carry a high risk. The average time between diagnosis and rupture is 16 months.

Ruptured abdominal aortic aneurysms are responsible for 1-1·5% of all deaths in men over the age of 65 in the Western World, with an incidence of 25-30/100 000 population.

Screening

Atheroma is associated with:

- Hypertension
- Diabetes
- Smoking
- Age
- Sex
- Hyperlipidaemia

Screening has recently been advocated to reduce the high incidence of ruptured aneurysms. The group at risk comprises men over 65, among whom there is a 2% prevalence of abdominal aneurysms >4 cm in diameter. Furthermore, a single ultrasound scan that shows an entirely normal aorta in a 60 year old man does not need to be repeated. Aneurysms <4 cm in diameter can usually be treated conservatively and followed up with six monthly ultrasound scans. Whether to operate on asymptomatic aneurysms <5 cm in diameter is controversial, but the risk of rupture was shown to be small in two recent population studies; the operation is indicated only if the aneurysms expand or start to cause symptoms.

Every undiagnosed aneurysm that ruptures must be seen as a failure of diagnosis and management

A screening programme for men over 60 would probably be cost effective because:

- The prevalence of aortic aneurysm in this group is 2%
- Ultrasonography is a simple, cheap, and accurate test
- The mortality associated with elective surgery is between 2% and 5%—and 90% if the aneurysm ruptures
- The life expectancy after successful aortic replacement is similar to that of age matched peers, the five year survival being more than 60%.

Presentation

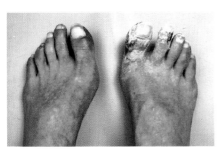

Atheromatous debris embolising to the feet causing discrete areas of necrosis, which may become infected. This patient had normal foot pulses.

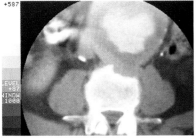

Erosion of the vertebral body by an aortic aneurysm.

Between 30% and 60% of abdominal aortic aneurysms are asymptomatic, and the commonest presenting symptom in the rest is low back pain caused by erosion of vertebral bodies. Erosion into the gastrointestinal tract (usually the third part of the duodenum) to form a primary aortoenteric fistula is rare, but carries a high mortality. Erosion into the vena cava is also rare and also carries a high mortality unless the diagnosis is made before operation. Distended superficial veins (which may be pulsatile), ankle oedema, cardiac failure, and raised central venous pressure in a patient with shock, together with a machinery murmur on abdominal auscultation, may alert the clinician to the diagnosis.

Pressure on peripheral nerves may cause pain in the groin or thigh and compression of adjacent veins causes ankle oedema. The aneurysmal sac can fill with thrombus and clot, and debris embolise distally to the legs, causing intermittent claudication or rest pain of sudden onset. Smaller emboli may occlude arterioles to the skin, causing small punctate areas of necrosis in the feet. Rarely occlusion of the mesenteric vessels causes left sided ischaemic colitis that presents with diarrhoea, which may be bloody. Organisms occasionally multiply in the atheroma or thrombus within the lumen of the aneurysm and the patient is likely to complain of non-specific symptoms such as weight loss, anorexia, and malaise.

Rarely, dense retroperitoneal fibrosis associated with an inflammatory aneurysm can occlude the ureters, causing hydronephrosis. Inflammatory aneurysms also cause severe backache that is associated with generalised malaise and anorexia. A high erythrocyte sedimentation rate is suggestive of this and computed tomography can usually confirm the diagnosis.

A pulsatile, expansile, abdominal mass is palpable in 80-90% of patients with abdominal aortic aneurysms. In thin patients smaller swellings (4-5 cm in diameter) may easily be felt. The diagnosis may be difficult in obese patients, however, and the size of the aneurysm is usually overestimated. If there is clinical doubt, ultrasonography is a simple and effective investigation. An aneurysm that is tender on palpation may indicate impending rupture, and urgent referral to a vascular surgeon is mandatory.

Investigation

Ultrasound beam

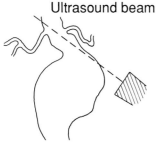

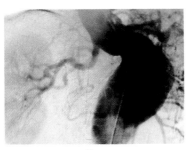

In an obese patient the ultrasound beam may not be transverse (left) thus erroneously suggesting a suprarenal aneurysm. The angiogram (right) shows the neck of the aneurysm to be well below the origin of the renal arteries.

The diagnosis is confirmed by ultrasound scanning, but inaccuracies of up to 8 mm must be expected. In addition, the neck of the aneurysm may also be incorrectly diagnosed as being above the renal arteries if an elongated tortuous aorta is twisted forwards.

Computed tomography of the abdomen provides more accurate anatomical information, but is more expensive. Arteriography is essential in a patient thought to have a thoracoabdominal aneurysm, abnormal renal function, or symptoms of distal occlusive disease, but if the aneurysm is uncomplicated it is probably unnecessary.

Operation and complications

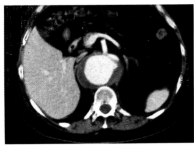

A computed tomogram with contrast showing a dissecting aneurysm occluding the origin of the superior mesenteric artery.

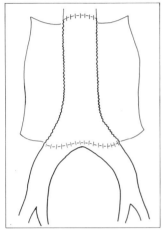

Tailoring the distal end to accommodate the origins of the iliac vessels may permit insertion of a tube graft for aneurysm repair.

It is important that the patient is warned before the operation of the small but pertinent risks associated with repair of an abdominal aortic aneurysm. The mortality is 2-5%, and a rare complication is paraplegia. A more usual problem is retrograde ejaculation, but true impotence is uncommon. Sigmoid ischaemia resulting in bloody diarrhoea or perforation may occur in 1-2% of patients; leg ischaemia may also arise from embolisation of the pultaceous debris in the aneurysmal sac.

The advances in anaesthetic and perioperative care during the past decade have made a great impact on results, but the operation has also been greatly simplified. In 60% of patients it is possible to insert a short Dacron tube rather than the more extensive aortobi-iliac or aortobifemoral grafts. Dissection of vessels can then be kept to a minimum and the graft laid inside the sac without disturbing surrounding structures.

Although prophylactic antibiotics are given at the time of operation, a small percentage of grafts still become infected. Patients may present with malaise, anorexia, weight loss, and fever. A gammacamera scan after injection of radiolabelled white cells may confirm the diagnosis, and computed tomography may show gas surrounding the graft. An aortoenteric fistula secondary to infection may present with haematemesis and melaena and should be suspected in a patient who has had an aneurysm repaired and who presents with such symptoms. Usually the blood loss into the gastrointestinal tract is intermittent, giving time for the diagnosis to be confirmed. Treatment is by removal of the graft together with revascularisation of the legs with bilateral axillofemoral grafts.

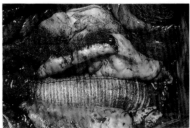

Aneurysmal sac is closed over the Dacron inlay tube graft.

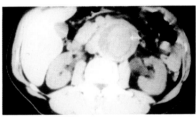

Thick walled inflammatory aneurysm (arrowed).

Thoracoabdominal aneurysms

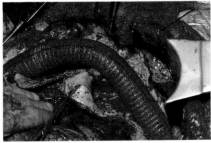

Extensive thoracoabdominal graft from level of left subclavian artery to the iliac bifurcation. Side holes of the graft are sewn directly to orifices of important visceral arteries.

Aortic aneurysms that include the origins of the visceral vessels used to be considered inoperable. Following recent encouraging reports from the United States, however, surgeons in some centres in the United Kingdom are repairing thoracoabdominal aneurysms, albeit with a higher mortality than after the repair of infrarenal aneurysms. In contrast to infrarenal aneurysms, thoracoabdominal aneurysms tend to be symptomatic. Most patients present with pain, although they may have other symptoms including dysphagia, dyspnoea, hoarse voice, and chronic cough. Careful preoperative assessment of cardiac, respiratory, and renal function is necessary and the risks of death, and visceral and spinal cord ischaemia, should be explained to the patient. Given the poor prognosis associated with these aneurysms, however, with only a quarter of the patients surviving two years, the results of surgery seem to be justified by survival rates of 60% at two years.

Conclusions

Only by early referral to a vascular surgeon can the appalling prognosis associated with rupture be avoided

Many aortic aneurysms are asymptomatic, so some form of screening is necessary to diagnose them. The most cost effective method is the routine abdominal examination of patients in the general practitioner's surgery, and two thirds of aneurysms >4 cm will be diagnosed by careful clinical examination. There are few absolute contraindications to operation. In particular, age is no bar.

TRAUMA

Averil O Mansfield, John H N Wolfe

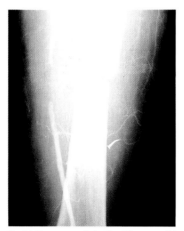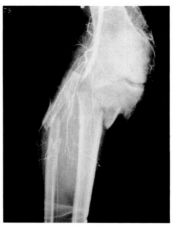

(Left) Fracture of shaft of femur with associated superficial femoral artery occlusion—easy to miss, but easy to repair. (Right) Comminuted fracture of tibia with popliteal artery occlusion—difficult to miss, and difficult to repair.

The diagnosis of vascular trauma is often either overlooked or delayed. Vascular injury should always be suspected in a patient who has had a road traffic accident and is shocked, or after any kind of penetrating injury such as a knife or gunshot wound. The most commonly missed injuries, however, are those associated with fractures of the long bones and dislocations. There is also an increasing number of iatrogenic injuries.

Types of injury

Types of injury

- Arterial
- Venous
- Associated fractures and nerve damage
- Arteriovenous fistulas
- False aneurysms

If an artery is completely transected the diagnosis is usually straightforward; the patient presents with haemorrhage or an expanding haematoma, or with an ischaemic extremity. Lacerations, dissections, and contusions may, however, be missed. A contused vessel may go into spasm, but this is nearly always associated with intimal damage and the risk of complete thrombosis, so the diagnosis of "spasm" should never be made unless more serious arterial injury has already been excluded. Arteriovenous fistulas may occur as a result of sharp penetrating injury.

Resuscitation

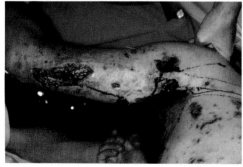

Lacerations of left arm due to bomb blast injury.

Haemorrhage declares itself; ischaemia is insidious and must be sought

It is essential that resuscitation should precede diagnosis in patients with multiple serious injuries. They are usually bleeding, pale, apprehensive, and short of breath. In a young, fit patient the blood pressure can be maintained by compensatory mechanisms; the patient may then collapse suddenly and the shock become irreversible.

Once an airway has been established, vital signs should be assessed and a rapid examination made. External bleeding can be controlled by direct pressure with a finger, a pressure dressing, or pressure on the arteries proximal to the bleeding point. Blind attempts to clamp bleeding vessels deep in the wound are dangerous and ineffective.

If the chest is injured the possibility of a haemopneumothorax must be considered before assisted ventilation has made the injury worse. Two large intravenous cannulas should be inserted, one for replacement of fluids and one for giving drugs.

If a patient is thought to have serious thoracic vascular injury, the vascular or cardiac surgeon should be consulted while the patient is being resuscitated in the emergency department. Injuries to limbs are usually seen first by orthopaedic surgeons, who should be trained to consider the possibility of vascular injury in every patient. If their suspicions are aroused the vascular surgeon should be called immediately so that priorities can be discussed.

Diagnosis

Misleading signs:

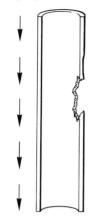

Transmitted pulse wave despite laceration.

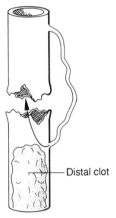

— Distal clot

Backbleeding through collateral vessel from distal artery, despite clot. Gentle balloon embolectomy should be done.

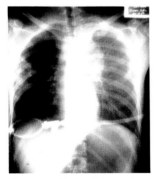

Upper mediastinal mass due to traumatic rupture of the aorta.

Referral to the radiology department should not delay treatment

---

Mechanism of injury

Penetrating injuries caused by stabbing or low velocity bullets are usually associated with damage that is confined to the track of the wound. In knife wounds it is useful to know the type and length of the knife, as this can alert the clinician to the possibility of an internal injury at a considerable distance from the surface wound (the spleen can be injured by a supraclavicular stab wound). High velocity bullets not only damage the neurovascular structures in their path, but also have a concussive effect as the energy dissipates and causes cavitation and damage to vessels some distance from the track. Shot gun pellets can also cause widespread damage as they are peppered through a wide area of tissue.

Blunt injuries—Motor vehicles are the main cause of accidental vascular trauma in Britain, and the two most common types are: (1) deceleration injuries to the major vessels and (2) those in association with fractured limbs.

Site of injury

Chest and abdomen—More than 15% of deaths after motor vehicle accidents are caused by rupture of the thoracic aorta. Less deceleration can produce partial rupture, so that examination of the femoral pulses and careful scrutiny of the chest radiograph to see if there is widening of the superior mediastinum may be crucial to the patient's survival.

Blunt injury may also fracture ribs and cause bleeding from the intercostal arteries into the pleural cavity. This causes surprisingly severe haemorrhage but is easy to treat.

Penetrating thoracic trauma may damage the intercostal arteries, the internal mammary artery, the superior and inferior vena cava, the pulmonary artery and vein, and the aorta or its major branches.

Arms and legs—Few patients die of vascular injuries of the arms or legs, but amputation or a painful, functionless limb are serious consequences of inadequate treatment. The amputation rate after major arterial injuries during world war II was 50%; it fell to 30% in the Korean war, and in civilian practice now is about 1·5%. The risk of losing a limb is greatest after blunt trauma, high velocity bullet wounds, or shotgun wounds at close range. This is largely because of the extent of tissue damage; wounds from knives and low velocity bullets seldom result in amputation but even these may have serious consequences if the popliteal artery is damaged.

After resuscitation the local injury should be assessed. Probes and fingers should not be inserted into the wound as this could dislodge clot and cause haemorrhage; bleeding is controlled best by direct pressure. Tourniquets should be avoided because they occlude inflow from collateral vessels and may increase the distal ischaemia. Blind clamping of the artery is dangerous because it can cause further damage to local vessels and may also damage adjacent structures, such as nerves.

Most injuries to limbs in Britain are associated with road traffic accidents—frequently to motor cyclists. In these patients the arterial injury may be concealed, and it cannot be emphasised enough that arterial spasm should not be diagnosed until there is firm evidence that there is no more serious damage to the artery. If the pulse is weak or absent, Doppler pressures should be measured. The presence of an arterial signal with a Doppler flowmeter may be misleading as this does not exclude damage to a major artery. A sphygmomanometer cuff should therefore be applied before the pressure is measured. If it is reduced compared with the opposite limb then arterial injury is likely. If there is proximal haematoma then late ischaemia may develop and a pulse oximeter is useful in monitoring the limb.

Investigation

A Doppler probe is valuable and should be readily available in the emergency department and wards. A chest radiograph is essential in the assessment of central injuries, and computed tomography may also help. The definitive investigation, however, is arteriography. This is useful in

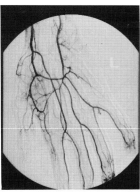

Thrombosis of digital arteries to the thumb caused by acute extension injury.

central injuries—firstly, because it helps to avoid unnecessary thoracotomy in a patient with serious injuries outside the thorax, and, secondly, because it can localise the site and extent of the arterial tear.

Some patients present with profound hypotension and a radiograph showing widening of the superior mediastinum, which suggests an extensive haematoma. These patients should not undergo aortography but should have exploration through a median sternotomy. A patient with a haemothorax associated with penetrating injuries or rib fractures probably has intercostal or internal mammary artery haemorrhage, and should also be operated on immediately.

Patients with subacute ischaemia of the limbs benefit from preoperative arteriography, but if the injury is acute the arteriogram should be done in the operating theatre.

Principles of repair

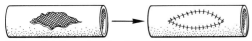

Vein patch for extensive laceration.

Obtain vein graft from an uninjured limb

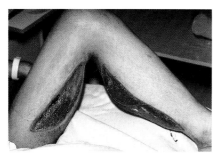

Calf and thigh fasciotomies after ischaemia caused by self administered intra-arterial injection of drugs.

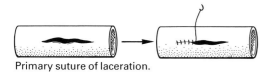

Primary suture of laceration.

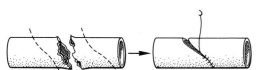

End to end anastomosis of healthy vessel.

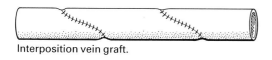

Interposition vein graft.

Control of haemorrhage, good access, debridement of surrounding contused tissues, and recognition of surrounding structures, particularly nerves, are the essential steps to successful repair of vascular injuries. Most patients with these injuries have normal arteries, which considerably improves the chances of a good result, but because the circulation has previously been normal there are no established collateral vessels, so that delay is disastrous.

Tears in arteries and veins can be closed primarily with a fine polypropylene suture. Great care must be taken to avoid stenosis of the vessel, and a vein patch is often required. When a vessel has been severed the same principles apply and it is essential that no anastomosis is made until the contused and damaged tissue has been removed. The two ends of the vessel can then be drawn together and a primary anastomosis done. The temptation is to stretch the vessels into apposition, but this will result in stenosis of the anastomosis and early failure. Again, a vein graft may be necessary and good results can be achieved by doing an oblique anastomosis. It is essential to obtain the vein graft from an uninjured limb because any further impairment of venous return may lead to problems later. Prosthetic grafts should not be used because of the risk of infection (they have been used in wartime to expedite treatment). The repair must then be covered with soft tissue, because secondary haemorrhage is very common in exposed grafts.

Fasciotomy is an important adjunct to any vascular repair and should be carefully considered in every case. It should always be done if the popliteal artery has been injured, or if there has been any delay in treatment. All four compartments should be decompressed either through removal of the middle segment of the fibula or through separate incisions.

Chest—Most major arterial injuries in the chest should be dealt with through a median sternotomy, which can be extended if necessary by a lateral incision to excise the clavicle or into one hemithorax.

Abdomen—Patients with penetrating wounds between the nipples and upper thigh may well have intra-abdominal vascular or visceral injuries: the key is early diagnosis. Blunt abdominal trauma usually causes either avulsion of vessels or intimal tears, which lead to secondary thrombosis. The most common vessels affected are the superior mesenteric artery, peripancreatic branches of the portal vein, and the left renal vein. Arterial tears are easily missed; for example, the renal artery may be thrombosed and the patient's only symptoms are some flank pain and haematuria. If the possibility is borne in mind the diagnosis should be made early and revascularisation carried out.

Injuries associated with fractures—For revascularisation of the leg to be successful the vessels must be repaired as soon as possible and the vascular anastomoses must be secure. The surgeon can therefore insert shunts into both artery and vein to restore flow and then allow the orthopaedic surgeon to stabilise the bony injury. This policy has been extremely successful in Belfast after "knee capping" injuries. On some occasions the orthopaedic surgeons may carry out rapid external fixation before the vascular repair, which is then stable. Manipulation of bone fragments and the limb after vascular repair damages the anastomosis and may result in early thrombosis. Contused nerves must be protected from damage and neurolysis is sometimes an essential part of revascularisation. If the vascular injury is associated with severe nerve injury, however, primary amputation may be the treatment of choice.

Venous injuries—Whenever possible venous injuries should be repaired at the same time as the arterial ones, and it was evident from the injuries in the Vietnam war that this was an important part of limb salvage. Certainly at the level of the popliteal fossa it is essential that there is adequate venous return to allow early decompression of the limb. Subsequently collateral vessels may develop, so that long term patency is probably less important. To repair larger veins it may be necessary to create a composite vein using either panels, or a spiral, of saphenous vein.

Limbs: soft tissue cover—It is essential that there is always closure of the soft tissues over the vessel. A vessel must always be covered by either muscle or skin, and if there is extensive loss of tissue, some form of flap may be necessary. Alternatively, uninjured muscle groups may be used to cover the repair.

Reimplantation—Excellent results are now being achieved from reimplantation of severed digits, hands, and arms. An amputated limb, or part of a limb, should therefore be kept clean and cool until a specialist opinion can be obtained.

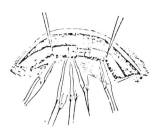

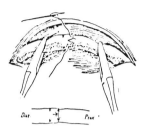

The first successful clinical end to end arterial anastomosis was performed in 1896 by J B Murphy in Chicago (from *Med Record* 1897;**51**:73).

Iatrogenic injuries

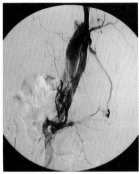

Arteriogram of right femoral arteriovenous fistula after cardiac catheterisation.

Many types of percutaneous catheter are now used for diagnosis and treatment so the number of iatrogenic injuries is increasing. There is a natural reticence to admit the degree of trauma and it is particularly in this group of patients that an erroneous diagnosis of spasm may be made. Catheters may cause dissections, perforations, arteriovenous fistulas, or false aneurysms. All these are easy to treat if they are recognised immediately. Haematomas around the brachial artery can be particularly insidious with apparently mild neurological complications. The correct treatment is to evacuate the haematoma and carry out neurolysis, because these nerve injuries may not resolve if they are left alone.

Reassessment

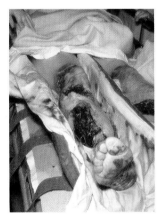
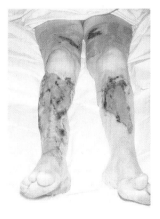

(Left) Fracture and extensive soft tissue injury after being run over by a truck. (Right) Good eventual result with full leg function.

Because most patients with vascular trauma are young and healthy the outlook is excellent providing that there has not been extensive associated damage and that the vascular repairs remain patent. Continuing assessment is essential, because an occult arterial injury or the need for fasciotomy may become apparent. Also, limbs in plaster that become painful may be ischaemic. Careful monitoring together with Doppler measurements or pulse oximetry, or both, keep the medical and nursing staff alert. The Doppler flowmeter must be used in conjunction with a sphygmomanometer cuff to measure pressure accurately.

A great deal can be lost very quickly in fit young patients unless we are alert to the possibilities of vascular injury and react appropriately.

CONVALESCENT PROBLEMS IN ARTERIAL SURGERY

Simon R G Smith, John H N Wolfe

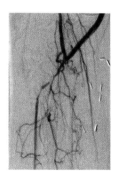

Successful bilateral femorocrural grafts have maintained this patient's independence, but the general practitioner must be aware of problems that may develop during convalescence.

Many of the patients who have problems after arterial reconstruction present to the general practitioner rather than to the vascular follow up clinic. Most can be managed satisfactorily at home, but a few require readmission to hospital. Serious problems are not common; modern vascular surgery should provide trouble free rehabilitation for many who would otherwise be incapacitated.

Early postoperative complications

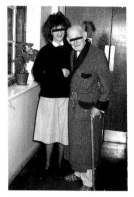

Progression of distal disease. The femoropopliteal graft remained patent but the distal popliteal artery had occluded and most of the flow was into the proximal popliteal artery.

Modern anaesthetic techniques such as epidural cannulation for pain relief enable rapid early recovery, particularly after aortic reconstruction. This—combined with the current pressure on surgical beds—has resulted in the earlier discharge of patients. On their return home the patients often complain of severe tiredness. This natural response to an operation requires explanation and reassurance. By the nature of the disease, however, myocardial ischaemia is always a threat and tiredness is one of the prodromal symptoms. Many patients are already receiving treatment for hypertension and angina before their operations, and procedures on the carotid, aortic, and renal arteries may alter the amount of antihypertensive treatment that they require, but optimal control may not be achieved until they are settled at home. Patients with unrecognised or latent disease—for example, diabetes—may be discharged taking new drugs.

Antiplatelet drugs are commonly prescribed for patients who have had reconstructions of small arteries. The rationale is that inhibition of platelet aggregation prevents their deposition on the surfaces of thrombogenic grafts and may help prevent neointimal hyperplasia. These drugs seem to help synthetic graft patency in the femoropopliteal segment but the evidence for increasing patency of autogenous vein is less convincing. After operations on the carotid artery lifelong treatment is often recommended, and aspirin 300 mg daily is effective in most patients.

After embolectomy aspirin is also indicated when the source of the embolus was a thrombus that occurred on the wall of a major vessel or after an infarct. When the origin was a fibrillating atrium the patient should be treated with anticoagulants unless there is a specific contraindication.

Smoking

There is now substantial evidence that continued smoking is associated with premature graft failure. Most patients manage to stop smoking while in hospital only to relapse at home. Encouragement to refrain should be directed not only towards the patient but also towards others in the family.

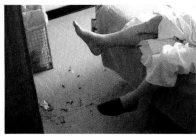

Some patients are unable to stop smoking even during the postoperative period of an operation to save a limb. This patient knocked his cigarette ends on to the floor in his haste to hide the evidence.

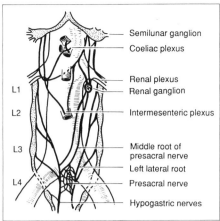

The autonomic nerves surrounding the abdominal aorta. Some damage to these (which is usually of no clinical consequence) is inevitable during aortic operations.

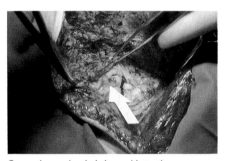

Slough of wound where the skin edge has been undermined.

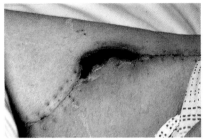

Sometimes dye is injected into the spaces between the toes. This is taken up by lymph and turns the vessels and nodes blue. They can then be avoided or ligated, thus avoiding lymph fistulas.

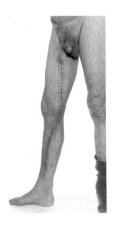

A long wound after femoroperoneal bypass grafting. Patients may be discharged from hospital before wounds are completely healed.

Activity

Walking is encouraged as this stimulates blood flow and venous return by the calf muscle pump. Once wounds have healed there is no danger of disrupting an anastomosis by normal convalescent activity. When resting the legs should be supported horizontally along their length until postoperative leg swelling has cleared.

Sexual function

Many patients with vascular disease will admit to having poor sexual function, and a few complain of it. The aetiology is complex. Impotence is a feature of aortoiliac disease and a few patients may benefit from internal iliac artery revascularisation. A deterioration in function after operation is common and requires sympathetic counselling. Operations on the aorta may damage the hypogastric and lumbar autonomic plexuses, resulting in retrograde or absent ejaculation or poor erection. Impotence can also follow loss of flow to the pudendal arteries, which is sometimes unavoidable.

Sexual activity can be resumed once the wounds are soundly healed (after about four to six weeks). Concern has been expressed about crossover femoral grafts that are placed subcutaneously over the pubis. Pressure on this area should be avoided to prevent thrombosis of the graft.

Wounds

By the time of discharge from hospital the access wounds for reconstruction should be healed. Minor amputation wounds may not be completely healed, but should be clean and granulating and require only dressings by a district nurse. Wounds that develop evidence of infection should have swabs taken for culture, especially if a synthetic graft (that is, anything except autologous vein) was used. The patient should be given a course of broad spectrum antibiotic—for example, erythromycin or cephradine—and referred back to the surgeon. Wound dehiscence and exposure of the graft requires immediate readmission to hospital.

Perigraft seroma (wound swelling)

Vascular surgical wounds, especially in the groin, are prone to developing lymphatic collections between the arterial bed and the skin. Most appear between the fifth and seventh postoperative days and commonly discharge clear, pale yellow fluid a few days later. The lymphatic fistula usually heals after treatment with bed rest and intensive nursing, but resuturing with the insertion of a closed suction drain is sometimes required. A lymphocele may develop after the patient has returned home, when the wound is well healed, but will usually settle if mobility is restricted to essential activity only. A perigraft seroma may develop around the length of a subcutaneous synthetic graft. The condition is generally benign and resolves with time, but early review by the surgeon is recommended. The temptation to aspirate these collections must be resisted because of the risk of infecting the graft. The late appearance of a collection may indicate infection of the graft.

Swelling of the lower limbs

Oedema of the lower limbs is common after femoropopliteal or more distal reconstructions and usually lasts for about six to eight weeks. The aetiology is not clear, but lymphatic obstruction, loss of subcutaneous venous channels, and reperfusion have been suggested. Oedema usually occurs when the long saphenous vein has been damaged, but it also occurs after bypasses with synthetic grafts. Taking the saphenous vein for use at other sites does not, however, cause oedema. Deep vein thrombosis is not the usual cause but should be considered, together with poor mobility when swelling develops late.

Anaesthetised areas

Incisions for exposing arteries—particularly the carotid, femoral, and popliteal arteries—may result in paresthesia, pain, or numbness because of injury to the cutaneous nerves. The effect is usually permanent and the patient should be reassured. Abnormal sensation indicates neuropraxia and recovery can be expected, though minor abnormalities may persist. Rarely, severe neuralgia may require carbamazepine 200 mg three times a day, but if this fails referral to a pain specialist for treatment such as transcutaneous stimulation should be considered.

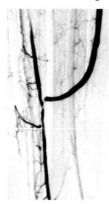

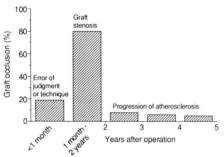

Stenosis developed a year after insertion of the graft at the distal anastomosis to the posterior tibial artery. This was successfully treated by balloon dilatation.

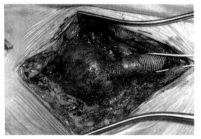

Most grafts that fail do so within the first year. Close surveillance is therefore indicated during this period.

Late complications

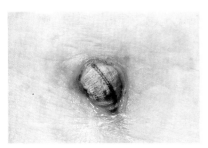

A false aneurysm between a Dacron graft and femoral artery. These usually result from failure of sutures, tension, or subclinical infection.

Axillofemoral Dacron grafts are placed subcutaneously, and breakdown of the wound may expose them. Exposed grafts almost inevitably become infected.

Failure of a graft

Failure of a graft results either in an acutely ischaemic limb (cool, pale, pulseless, and painful, becoming anaesthetised and discoloured) or in a return to the patient's preoperative state. Failure within a month after operation is usually secondary to a technical problem. The patient should be readmitted to hospital urgently. If intervention takes place early enough many grafts can be salvaged, but delay results in a lost graft. Subcutaneous grafts can be palpated easily and the patient or a relative should be taught to monitor the pulse in the graft daily so that they can report its disappearance or the sudden return of symptoms.

Failure between one month and a year after operation is commonly the result of stenotic changes in the graft or obstruction of anastomoses by myointimal hyperplasia. Despite great efforts in recent years directed towards predicting failure by non-invasive monitoring, grafts continue to fail unexpectedly during the early months. Measurements of pressures by Doppler scanning with or without a stress test and, more recently, by duplex Doppler scanning have been used. Pressure studies are not good predictors of failure, as important stenoses may be present without a measurable drop in pressure. Duplex scanning can reliably detect stenoses of 20% or more of the luminal area, but it is not yet clear whether all stenoses endanger the patency of the graft. Intensive regular monitoring (every two months to six months) is not always feasible, and grafts may deteriorate between reviews. The development of even mild symptoms is a reliable indicator of trouble; patients should therefore report if symptoms develop so that early reassessment can be arranged. They should not wait for the routine outpatient appointment.

After a year failure of a graft is usually the result of progression of disease. At five years about 90% of aortofemoral vein grafts and 70% of femoropopliteal grafts are patent.

Thrombosis of a reconstructed vessel

Late thrombosis occurs when flow through a reconstructed vessel is critically reduced at the inflow or outflow point, usually by progression of the disease. Segments that have been cleared by endarterectomy may also restenose. Dacron grafts elongate with time and kinking may cause an appreciable stenosis. Rarely, the neointima delaminates. Acute ischaemia requires urgent admission to hospital, though often there is spontaneous improvement. Reduction of flow is usually progressive, however, and an adequate collateral circulation develops in parallel. As a result reconstructions fail without a noticeable change in performance and may not be discovered until a routine review. Under such circumstances no action may be necessary.

False aneurysm

A false aneurysm—a pulsatile sac without a true vascular wall—results from a small leak through a suture line and is usually caused by degenerative change; between 3% and 5% of prosthetic grafts are affected. The groin is the most common site, but any suture line between graft and vessel— including around the synthetic patches that have been used to close vessels after endarterectomy—may be affected. The sac grows slowly and ultimately may thrombose, discharge emboli, or rupture causing haemorrhage. When a false aneurysm is detected an early outpatient review should be arranged so that the surgeon may assess the need for correction. Pain, tenderness, and increasing size are indications for action.

Graft infection

Infection is the most serious complication of vascular grafts and threatens both life and limb. It occurs in 1% to 2% of prosthetic grafts, most commonly in the groin, and may appear at any time. Pain, low grade fever, septic embolic foci, and haemorrhage all suggest infection. Clinical awareness is paramount as the diagnosis is difficult to confirm.

The causes of infection include contamination during insertion of the graft, erosion of adjacent gut by the graft, penetrating injury, or bloodborne inoculation. It is therefore important that patients with prosthetic grafts are given appropriate antibiotic prophylaxis during any subsequent invasive procedures, particularly on the gastrointestinal or genitourinary tracts.

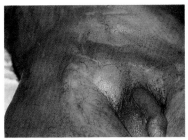

This patient had an abscess in the right groin and an abscess from an aortoenteric fistula secondary to an infected graft. He survived after removal of the infected aortic graft and bilateral axillofemoral grafting.

Conclusion

When there is doubt about a problem a prompt telephone discussion between general practitioner and surgeon will help to resolve it.

Patients with suspected graft infection require urgent assessment in hospital.

Aortoenteric fistula

The possibility of an aortoenteric fistula must be considered in any patient with an aortic graft who presents with a gastrointestinal haemorrhage. A warning bleed usually occurs before a catastrophic haemorrhage. Emergency admission to hospital is required and—in the absence of any obvious cause—exploratory laparotomy should be planned with the expectation of having to remove the graft and restore the blood supply with bilateral axillofemoral grafts.

This article has discussed the complications of peripheral arterial reconstruction, but the principles apply equally to reconstructions of other arteries such as carotid, renal, and mesenteric arteries. Arterial reconstructions are complex but they enable an independent mobile existence for many patients. The common problems are the most simple to manage. With prompt action the more serious problems can usually be resolved satisfactorily, leading to restoration of function.

The histogram is based on data derived from Brewster *et al*, *Arch Surg* 1983;**118**:1104. We thank Mr A V Pollock for the picture of colour lymphography.

LATE COMPLICATIONS OF ARTERIAL GRAFTS

P Rutter, John H N Wolfe

Five main types of complication

- The graft blocks (**ischaemia**)
- Late disruption around the anastomosis (**true and false aneurysms**)
- The graft sends off showers of thrombi (**emboli**)
- The graft becomes colonised with micro-organisms (**infection**)
- An intra-abdominal graft may erode adjacent viscera (usually **aortoenteric fistulas**)

Most complications associated with the insertion of vascular grafts occur after the patient has been discharged from hospital, and so are presented firstly to the general practitioner.

Saphenous nerve damage is relatively common and may result in paraesthesia or numbness on the lower medial thigh. Femoral nerve damage is much less common but more serious, with weakness of the knee flexor muscles. The damage is usually reversible if it has been caused by retraction of the nerve during dissection. Carbamazepine or transcutaneous nerve stimulation may be useful for patients with severe unrelenting symptoms, but in most people symptoms resolve rapidly and reassurance is all that is required.

Ischaemia

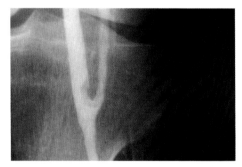

Lower end of PTFE graft anastomosed to the popliteal artery showing stenosis developing at the heel.

The sudden occlusion of a graft should easily be recognised by both doctor and patient. There must be no delay in referral back to the surgeon, particularly if the limb is viable, because a longstanding occlusion can rarely be unblocked; early treatment is the essence of success. A cool, pale, pulseless leg with full movement and early muscle tenderness requires urgent intervention.

The degree of ischaemia that occurs after a graft blocks depends both on the collateral supply and the extent to which the native artery is occluded. Early treatment is essential because delay may result in the loss of the graft and often of the limb as well.

Causes

At least 10% of grafts are occluded by five years. The rate increases the more distal the graft, and if synthetic materials are used; more than half of all femorodistal grafts are occluded by five years.

If the cause of occlusion is surgical error (either in operative technique or patient selection) it will happen early—within 30 days of the operation. If a graft occludes between one and 18 months of operation the reason is usually narrowing of the lumen of the graft by neointimal hyperplasia, which is proliferation of smooth muscle and deposition of connective tissue in the intima of the graft. Most occlusions that happen more than two years after operation are caused by progression of the atheromatous disease in the native vessels.

Prevention

One recent large study showed that stopping smoking was a more important factor than drug manipulation in increasing survival of grafts. Nevertheless, drugs have a role, particularly in patients with a narrow distal graft, and many patients are discharged from hospital taking either warfarin or aspirin.

Serial non-invasive surveillance of infrainguinal bypass grafts is now recommended. Doppler techniques can identify grafts at risk by showing low flow in the graft and by localising stenoses within the graft and early detection and treatment can significantly increase long term patency.

Diagnosis

Recurrence of the symptoms that were present before the operation suggests occlusion of the graft. For example, in a patient with claudication who initially has an improved walking distance but then returns to the preoperative distance or less.

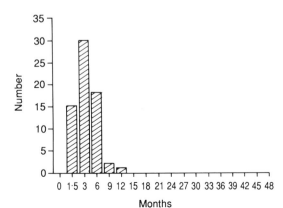

Number of grafts that develop new stenoses according to time after surgery.

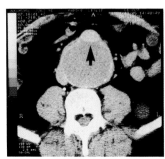

Early stages of graft thrombolysis with streptokinase. Note that patency has been achieved but lysis of residual clot remains necessary.

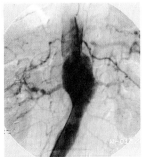

Right lower leg showing incisions for "jump graft" from vein graft with distal stenosis to the posterior tibial artery at the ankle.

Patients usually present with rest pain but painless gangrene of the extremities with serious tissue loss is seen too often.

Physical examination should concentrate both on the tissues and the arteries supplied by the graft. If the collateral arterial supply is adequate for the tissues at rest then no skin or neuromuscular changes are seen. If the occlusion is causing critical ischaemia then the limb is cold, becomes pallid when it is raised, and capillary return is slow.

Before examining the pulses both in the graft and distal to it, it is essential to know what happened after the operation. The discharge summary should state whether the pulses were palpable or could be located only with a Doppler probe.

The pulse can usually be felt in a functioning subcutaneous vein graft so a patient may have a functioning graft (associated with severe distal atheromatous disease) but be without a palpable peripheral pulse. Synthetic grafts are not usually pulsatile.

Education of the patient

Patients should be told to return to the vascular surgeon immediately if there is a sudden change in symptoms. Too often they present late, when the graft is irreversibly blocked. They should also be taught to monitor their own grafts or distal pulses if these can easily be felt.

Management

The first consideration is the condition of the limb. Irreversible ischaemia or infarction means that immediate amputation is the only option. Misguided attempts at revascularisation may result in fatal cardiac or renal toxicity. On the other hand the combination of graft failure and an unthreatened leg may not require further intervention.

If intervention is required it must be early, because the success rates of simpler methods of graft salvage (surgical thrombectomy or angiographic thrombolysis) decrease with delay. Graft failure that is recognised immediately responds well to thrombolytic agents such as streptokinase or tissue plasminogen activator. The local stenosis can then be recognised and a localised operation carried out. Thrombolytic drugs should not be used, however, if the limb is acutely ischaemic with no movement or sensation and muscle that is probably dead. Such a limb requires immediate thrombectomy and, under these circumstances, intraoperative arteriography should identify the cause of failure and help plan the revascularisation.

True and false aneurysms

Arteriogram showing the aneurysm of aorta that has developed 10 years after insertion of the original infrarenal graft.

Computed tomogram showing false aneurysm of abdominal aorta between abdominal aorta and aortic graft (arrowed).

Causes

Anastomotic aneurysms result from a partial or total separation of the anastomosis between the artery and the vascular graft, which are then connected only by a fibrous capsule. They arise after breakdown of the suture line between the graft and the arterial wall, either because the graft or the sutures fail or because the arterial wall is destroyed by infection. Improvements in modern sutures and grafts mean that most aneurysms are now caused either by technical errors such as excessive graft tension or poor placement of sutures, or by infection of the graft. Occult infection is now appreciated as a more common cause of graft aneurysms than was previously supposed.

The incidence of anastomotic aneurysm has been estimated at between 1% and 4% and the most common site is the lower end of an aortobifemoral graft.

Diagnosis

Most anastomotic aneurysms are asymptomatic, although some may cause symptoms by pressing on local structures.

If the aneurysm is superficial it can be palpated easily. A chronic, non-pulsatile swelling at the site of an anastomosis is more likely to be a collection of lymph (lymphocele).

Management

Anastomotic aneurysms should be repaired, and usually a short segment of bypass graft is required, but the operation may be unexpectedly complex. Although small aneurysms can initially be treated conservatively, the risk of rupture increases as they expand.

Late complications of arterial grafts
Emboli

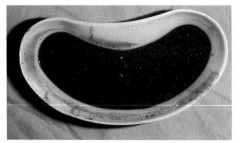

Dish containing blood from initial flush of an aortic graft. This shows a considerable amount of debris that might embolise to the legs.

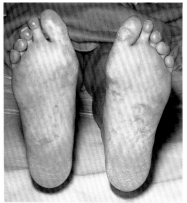

Feet showing postoperative cutaneous emboli.

Infection

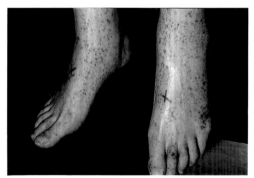

Petechial emboli in patient with an aortic graft infected with staphylococci.

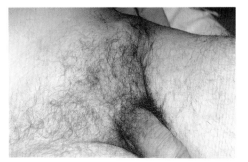

Left groin abscess: the herald sign of graft infection.

Most emboli are thromboembolic and are more common in large calibre proximal grafts, particularly those inserted for aneurysmal disease. Septic emboli are less common and originate from prosthetic grafts. Most emboli from grafts occur immediately after the operation, and the incidence from grafts that have been in place for more than a month is low.

Diagnosis

The symptoms depend on the site at which the embolus lodges distal to the graft and on the size of the embolus. Patients with emboli to intra-abdominal organs such as the gut or kidneys may present with either pain or organ failure. More commonly the emboli lodge in the limbs and cause symptoms varying from the pain of severe ischaemia to small areas of skin infarction.

Acute ischaemia caused by an embolus occluding a major vessel can result in the classic "five Ps": pale, painful, pulseless, paraesthesia, and perishing (with cold). Small emboli may lodge in the skin and cause characteristic clusters of petechial lesions.

Management

Balloon embolectomy is the best treatment for thromboemboli as the older organised clot and sections of pseudointima that make up most of these emboli do not respond well to thrombolytic drugs. But as showers of emboli also lodge in the more distal vessels adjunctive thrombolysis may help. In some cases further bypass is necessary to vessels beyond the occlusions. Septic emboli must be treated by removal of the infected graft and treatment with antibiotics.

One of the main drawbacks of modern prosthetic grafts is their susceptibility to infection, and manufacturers are currently attempting to protect the material with antibiotic coating. Infections occurring more than 30 days after operation may be difficult to detect because there may be few organisms of low virulence. The consequences can, however, be disastrous.

When the graft is within the abdomen the incidence of infection is low. If the graft extends into the groin, however, the incidence increases (to 2-3%), particularly if there has been a collection of blood, serous fluid, or lymph.

Causes

The most common cause of infection is contamination of the graft at the time of operation, but other sources of infection are contaminated blood and lymph. Femoral incisions necessitating disruption of lymphatic channels are particularly susceptible if there is distal infection or gangrene. Any patient with a prosthetic graft who develops bacteraemia or lymphadenitis should therefore be treated promptly with antibiotics to minimise the risk of colonisation of the graft.

Cellular adherence and turnover on a prosthetic graft do not cease, so that any transient bacteraemia can lead to late graft infection. Suitable prophylaxis should therefore be arranged for any invasive procedure such as tooth extraction or cystoscopy.

Diagnosis

There may be systemic signs such as fever, but rigors are uncommon. There are often no local findings but non-specific malaise in a patient with a prosthetic graft should arouse suspicion of infection.

The infection may drain through a sinus in the wound. If the graft is placed subcutaneously palpation may indicate the presence of an aneurysm in the inflammatory mass. Skin petechiae distal to the graft are a rare but diagnostic finding.

No investigation shows both good specificity and sensitivity. A raised erythrocyte sedimentation rate is almost always present but is non-specific. The white cell count is raised only if the infection is caused by virulent organisms. Once the patient is in hospital computed tomography and angiography are usually carried out, but scanning of indium labelled white cells is the most sensitive test at present.

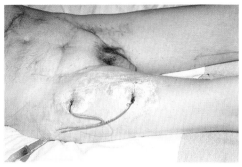

Localised graft infection in the right groin treated with continuous gentamicin infusion.

Management

The principles of management are removal of the infected graft, debridement of infected tissue, and treatment with antibiotics. Immediate revascularisation with a new graft should be avoided, but when it is essential (such as after removal of an aortic graft) the graft should be extra-anatomical—for example, axillofemoral—to avoid the bed of the infected graft. Under specific circumstances irrigation of an infected prosthesis with antibiotic solution may be effective.

Aortoenteric fistulas

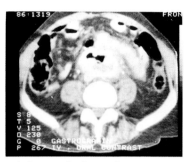

Diagnostic free gas in the aortic sac on computed tomography. The patient had an episode of melaena, giving the diagnosis of aortoenteric fistula.

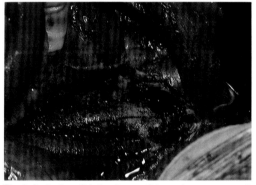

The infected graft lying in small bowel contents and the clot from the aortoenteric fistula.

Most aortoenteric fistulas present months or years after the initial operation and the incidence is between 0·4% and 4%. When the centre of the graft erodes into the gut, digestion of the fibrous tissue surrounding the graft causes slow seepage of blood into the intestine. If the graft/artery suture line breaks down, however, there is a risk of exsanguinating haemorrhage. The areas of intestine most commonly affected are the distal duodenum and the duodenojejunal flexure.

Diagnosis

Gastrointestinal bleeding, whatever the volume, in a patient with an aortic graft should raise the suspicion of a connection between the graft and the small intestine. The bleeding may be occult or modest, the so called "herald" bleed. An episode of melaena in these patients is therefore due to an aortoenteric fistula until proved otherwise.

The anastomotic aneurysm that causes the bleed is rarely palpable and the fistulous connection is often in the fourth part of the duodenum or upper jejuneum, beyond the range of the gastroduodenoscope. Endoscopy is useful, however, because a source of serious bleeding in the stomach or proximal duodenum is excluded. Computed tomography may show an anastomotic aneurysm or collections of fluid and air around the graft, indicating infection.

Management

The gut must be repaired and the graft removed. The aortic stump and distal vascular tree are oversewn, and viability of the lower limb is maintained by extra-anatomical axillofemoral grafts, which avoid the infected abdominal cavity.

THROMBOSIS AND PULMONARY EMBOLISM

N F G Hopkins, John H N Wolfe

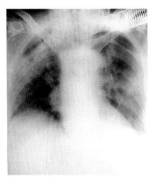

Chest radiograph showing
pulmonary embolism.

Risk factors

Immobility
Age >40 years
History of deep vein thrombosis
Varicose veins
Obesity
Malignant disease
Pregnancy
The puerperium
Oral contraception
Surgery
Trauma
Myocardial infarction
Heart failure
Polycythaemia
Thrombocytopenia
Connective tissue disease
Congenital coagulation disorders

It is difficult to assess the incidence of deep vein thrombosis accurately and the figures that are available are probably underestimates. By using objective diagnostic techniques, however, deep vein thromboses are detectable in 25-35% of patients after operations, and in 20-50% of patients after myocardial infarctions or strokes. Pulmonary embolism kills 1/10 000 men and 1·5/10 000 women every year in England and Wales.

Venous thrombi are initiated by changes in the coagulation mechanisms of the blood, damage to the endothelial lining of blood vessels, and by reduction in blood flow—the three components of Virchow's triad that was first described in 1846. A fourth component should now be added—the fibrinolytic state of the patient.

Certain factors alter the balance of these mechanisms; immobility is the most important (particularly if it lasts for four days or longer), and a previous deep vein thrombosis will have caused intimal scarring and venous pooling, and therefore will predispose to further thrombosis. Malignant disease may result in the production of procoagulant material or reduced fibrinolytic activity. Operations are associated with many of the factors— the trauma activating the clotting factors and the stasis occurring during the procedure and recovery period. The extent and duration of the operation also influence the degree of risk. The type of procedure influences the probability of local damage to vessels, which is particularly common in operations on the lower limb and in the pelvic region. Some patients are predisposed to deep vein thrombosis because of deficiencies in blood and tissue factors including antithrombin III, protein C, protein S, and plasminogen activator—a substance released from vein walls and blood, and vital for the activation of the fibrinolytic system. Conversely, high concentrations of plasminogen inhibitor have also been detected in patients with iliofemoral thromboses.

Many patients will have more than one risk factor, and it is important to realise that the overall risk is the product rather than the sum of the individual factors; thus the risk is greatly increased by the coexistence of two or more factors.

Prophylaxis

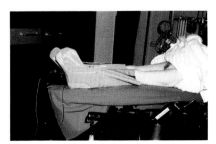

Single chamber intermittent pneumatic
compression boots.

Prophylaxis is probably the most important aspect when considering thromboembolic disease; it is directed towards reducing venous stasis and combating the changes in the blood that promote coagulation.

Venous stasis may be reduced by physical methods, many of which are simple. For patients having operations they include careful positioning of the patient on the operating table to avoid pressure on the calves, avoiding restriction of venous outflow, and early ambulation after the operation.

External compression by elastic stockings is an inexpensive and safe method of increasing venous velocity but it is important that the compression is graduated. Intermittent pneumatic compression with a single or multichamber device and electrical calf muscle stimulation also improve venous flow during operation.

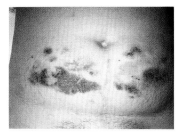

Subcutaneous bruising after prolonged treatment with subcutaneous heparin. Patients who develop such problems should be given the injections into their backs.

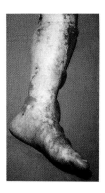

Idiopathic thrombocytopenic reaction to heparin resulting in ischaemia of the leg.

Presentation and diagnosis

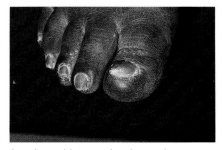

A patient with extensive deep vein thrombosis may present with venous gangrene.

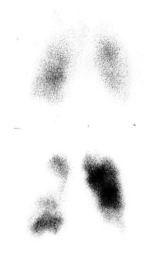

Ventilation and perfusion lung scans showing "mismatch" in right upper lobe.

Of the pharmacological methods available, low dose heparin is the most widely used and thoroughly evaluated. The heparin is given subcutaneously in a dose of 5000 units at 8 or 12 hourly intervals starting before the operation and continuing until the patient is ambulant. A large multicentre trial showed significant reductions in the incidence of deep vein thrombosis and pulmonary embolism when patients receiving this regimen were compared with a control group receiving no prophylaxis. The only complication is wound haematoma, and this makes the method unacceptable for neurosurgical operations and operations in which a lot of dissection is necessary. Results have also been disappointing in the high risk group of patients having hip prostheses inserted, but low molecular weight heparins may be more effective.

Dihydroergotamine causes venous vasoconstriction thus increasing blood flow, and trials have shown that this may be useful when combined with heparin given subcutaneously. Side effects are rare but skin gangrene has been reported, and the drug should be avoided in patients with myocardial infarction, vasospastic disorders, peripheral arterial disease, or sustained hypotension.

Dextran is also effective. Its use does, however, require the intravenous infusion of 500-1000 ml of fluid before and on at least alternate days after operation. This is cumbersome and may interfere with fluid balance; furthermore, complications associated with bleeding are common.

In summary, a prophylactic regimen for a particular patient should be adopted after balancing the degree of risk against the potential complications of the prophylaxis. All patients at risk should wear graduated compression stockings and heparin should be given subcutaneously to patients at particularly high risk.

Deep vein thrombosis

The appearance of common clinical signs of deep vein thrombosis should arouse suspicion, particularly if the patient is in a high risk group, but other conditions may present in similar ways. Fever and tachycardia are of little diagnostic importance; less than half of the patients with local tenderness or Homan's sign have deep vein thrombosis; and only half the limbs in which there are clinical signs below the knee contain thrombi. Conversely, more than half of all deep vein thromboses are clinically silent and are detected only by screening.

The diagnosis should therefore always be confirmed before treatment is started. Ultrasound scanning will show only occlusive thrombi, and is unhelpful if the thrombus is confined to the calf. Venography is the standard technique and provides anatomical information, an estimate of the age of the thrombus, and a measure of whether it is fixed to the wall of the vessel or floating free. Impedance plethysmography is an accurate, non-invasive diagnostic test for thrombosis at or proximal to the popliteal vein, but false positive results may occur in patients who have arterial insufficiency.

Scanning the uptake of fibrinogen labelled with iodine-125 is a sensitive test, especially for early thrombosis confined to the calf, and permits serial analysis on consecutive days. Unfortunately this test is suitable only for screening, because preparation includes blocking the uptake of iodine by the thyroid.

Pulmonary embolism

Pulmonary embolic disease also presents in various ways depending on the extent and age of the embolism. It can be classified as "massive" (more than half of the pulmonary arterial tree is occluded) or "minor," and as "acute" (of less than 48 hours' duration), "subacute," or "chronic." Acute massive embolism results in sudden reduction in cardiac output and circulatory collapse. Patients with subacute massive embolism and chronic thromboembolic disease are rare and present with increasing dyspnoea, pulmonary hypertension, and right heart failure.

Acute minor embolism is most commonly seen, and may warn of an impending fatal embolus.

Minor embolism does not cause serious haemodynamic disturbance but patients present with pleuritic pain, haemoptysis, and signs such as pleural rub, effusion, or collapse/consolidation. The diagnosis may be difficult soon after an operation and if there is pre-existing cardiorespiratory disease. The

Thrombosis and pulmonary embolism

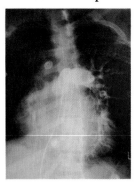

Pulmonary angiogram showing pulmonary embolism.

Management

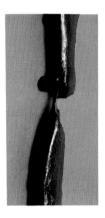

Thrombus removed at thrombectomy showing site of valve.

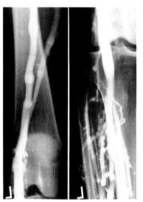

Venogram from the same patient taken one year later showing competent deep venous system with no damage to valves.

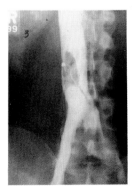

Greenfield inferior vena cava filter containing a clot, and with a clot extruding from it.

chest radiograph may show pulmonary opacities, elevation of the diaphragm, effusion, atelectasis, and — in larger emboli — areas of oligaemia. Perfusion lung scans show deficits where the artery is obstructed, but in patients with coexistent respiratory disease simultaneous ventilation and perfusion scars are essential to see if there is normal ventilation in the areas of oligaemia. The $S_1 Q_3 T_3$ electrocardiographic pattern is pathognomonic of a large pulmonary embolus and reflects right heart strain, but it is present in less than half of patients with large emboli. Changes in blood gas tensions are non-specific but may offer a guide to the extent of the embolism. Pulmonary arteriography is the definitive investigation, but is indicated only in critically ill patients to confirm the diagnosis so that the correct treatment may be started.

The three main aims of treatment of deep vein thrombosis are to prevent extension of the thrombus, to reduce the risk of embolism, and to avoid the long term complications of the postphlebitic limb. The treatment will depend on the site and extent of the thrombus, which should be confirmed objectively. In about 80% of cases the thrombus is confined to the calf veins, but it may propagate into the veins of the popliteal fossa, thigh, and pelvis. In some cases the thrombus arises in the iliofemoral segment, and may extend distally.

If the thrombi are small and confined to the calf treatment should be conservative and comprise limb exercise in bed, raising the foot of the bed, and wearing elastic compression stockings. For more extensive thrombi the patient should be given heparin intravenously to maintain the activated partial thromboplastin time at 2-3 times the normal value. Recent studies, however, have suggested that calcium heparin given subcutaneously may be equally effective in preventing propagation of thrombi. Oral anticoagulant drugs should be started at the same time and continued for 8-12 weeks. Warfarin is given in a loading dose of 20-30 mg over 3 days and then daily, the dose being adjusted to maintain a prothrombin time of 2·0-3·0 times the normal value by using international reference thromboplastin.

Thrombolytic treatment with streptokinase, urokinase, or tissue plasminogen activator should be reserved for more extensive thrombosis. It is most effective when the thrombus is reasonably fresh and only partially occlusive, and may salvage deep veins — thus reducing the incidence of postphlebitic changes. These agents require careful monitoring, however, and carry a greater risk of haemorrhage than simple anticoagulant drugs. Furthermore, streptokinase may (rarely) cause an anaphylactic reaction, and urokinase — which does not have this drawback — is extremely expensive.

Thrombectomy should be reserved for cases of extensive proximal thrombosis in which anticoagulants are contraindicated or the viability of the limb is threatened. The temporary construction of an arteriovenous fistula, or intermittent pneumatic compression, have been used to maintain venous patency with some success.

Interruption of vena caval flow should be reserved for patients who develop emboli while receiving anticoagulant drugs; those in whom anticoagulation is contraindicated; and, possibly, those with life threatening, large, proximal, non-adherent thrombi. Early techniques required major operations and resulted in a high incidence of extensive distal thrombosis, peripheral oedema, and postphlebitic change. Modern equipment such as the Greenfield and Gunther filters do not have these disadvantages because they permit continued caval flow and may be inserted through the jugular vein with the patient under local anaesthesia.

The management of minor pulmonary emboli is aimed at preventing recurrence or extension. Anticoagulant drugs should be prescribed.

Patients with massive established emboli should initially be resuscitated. Pulmonary arteriography should be considered to confirm the diagnosis and assess the extent of the embolus. If resuscitation has been successful and the patient is stable, treatment is by thrombolytic drugs; if not, pulmonary embolectomy offers the only hope of survival.

The illustration of idiopathic thrombocytopenia was first published in *Surgery (Oxford)* 1987;**1**:967-71 and is reproduced by kind permission of The Medicine Group (UK).

DEEP VENOUS INSUFFICIENCY AND OCCLUSION

N F G Hopkins, John H N Wolfe

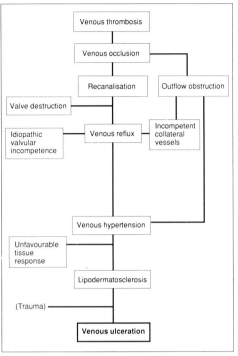

Sequence of events leading to venous ulceration.

Pulmonary embolus is a serious complication of deep vein thrombosis but deep venous insufficiency or occlusion, or both, are much more common long term problems and many venous ulcers occur each year, putting strains on both the work force and health service resources. It has long been recognised that deep vein thrombosis is usually followed by recanalisation of the veins and that this process results in destruction of the venous valves, which in turn results in deep venous insufficiency. Failure to recanalise results in chronic venous occlusion with the development of a collateral circulation that is also without valves. Either event has a deleterious effect on the function of the calf muscle pump, resulting in high venous pressure in the leg and foot even during exercise. This is the fundamental abnormality that results in a postphlebitic limb with venous ulceration or venous claudication. In addition, some patients have a congenital absence of competent valves without evidence of previous thrombosis.

Diagnosis

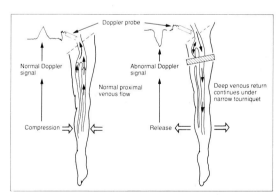

Detection by Doppler ultrasonography of deep venous insufficiency at the common femoral vein.

Clinical

A history of deep vein thrombosis should be sought together with a history of disorders associated with a high incidence of thrombosis, such as operations on the pelvis or hip, or a complicated obstetric course. Venous claudication is characterised by severe "bursting" pain in the calf after exercise. Because the superficial collateral vessels are sometimes important, elastic stockings—which compress these veins—may sometimes exacerbate the symptoms. The pain is relieved by rest but—in contrast to arterial claudication—is often improved by elevation of the limb.

Physical signs associated with deep venous disease include swelling; the appearance of superficial collateral veins; and thickening, induration, and pigmentation of the subcutaneous tissues in the gaiter area (lipodermatosclerosis). The skin itself may be thickened and sclerotic, and it may be ulcerated or show the scars of healed ulcers.

On examination of the superficial veins there may be varicosities, and the Trendelenburg tourniquet test will fail to control venous reflux because of the multiple sites of incompetence between the deep and superficial venous systems. Perthes' test should be used to see if there is deep venous obstruction. A tourniquet is applied below the knee to occlude the superficial collateral veins. If the deep veins are also occluded the patient will experience pain on exercise.

Doppler ultrasonography

Deep venous obstruction may be detected as described in the article on thrombosis and pulmonary embolism. Deep venous insufficiency may be

Deep venous insufficiency and occlusion

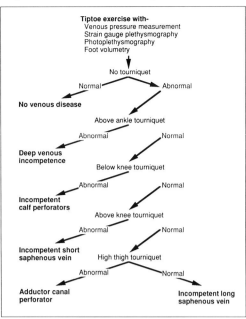

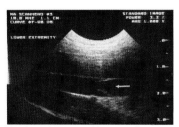

Quantitative testing for venous incompetence.

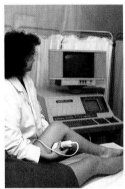

Duplex Doppler assessment of venous system.

Duplex ultrasound image of veins with cusps open.

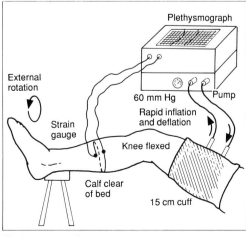

Plethysmography.

diagnosed with a simple hand held Doppler scanner. The test takes only one or two minutes to do: the patient is examined standing, and the probe placed over the common femoral vein at the groin. After placement of a narrow, high thigh tourniquet to occlude the superficial veins, and with the patient bearing weight on the opposite limb, the venous signal is confirmed when the patient takes a deep breath; it can be enhanced by squeezing the patient's calf. When the pressure on the calf is released there should be no signal, as competent valves prevent reflux of blood down the limb. Should a signal last longer than a second, deep venous insufficiency is present. This reflux signal may be confirmed by the patient carrying out a Valsalva manoeuvre.

The test can also be done by examining the popliteal vein with a tourniquet placed at the level of the upper calf; there should be no signal on release of pressure on the calf.

Although they are less important, the posterior tibial veins may be examined with a tourniquet above the ankle; when pressure is applied to the calf there should be no signal, but there should be an enhanced venous signal when the pressure is released.

In specialist laboratories duplex Doppler scanning may be used to study the functions of venous valves by imaging the movement of valve cusps during both respiration and the Valsalva manoeuvre. The Valsalva manoeuvre snaps the valve cusps together. Bidirectional flow in incompetent systems is detected by audible signals and spectral analysis.

Direct measurement of venous pressure

This remains the most established method of assessing the function of calf muscle pumps. A fine needle is inserted into a vein on the dorsum of the foot and connected to a pressure transducer and thence to a pen recorder. Pressure is recorded with the patient standing at rest, and during and after a period of standardised exercise—usually exercises moving on to "tip toe" once a second for 20 seconds. In normal subjects a fall in venous pressure of 50-90% of the resting pressure is seen with a return to resting pressure within 20-40 seconds of stopping the exercise. Deep venous obstruction results in a rise in pressure on exercise, but more commonly deep venous insufficiency shows a varied but reduced fall in pressure accompanied by a more rapid return to resting pressure. This standard exercise regimen is done both with and without tourniquets to occlude the superficial veins. If initial testing gives abnormal results but the placing of tourniquets returns calf pump function to normal the abnormality lies within the superficial venous system and will be suitable for operation. Should the test results remain abnormal when the tourniquets are used, then deep venous insufficiency is present.

Plethysmography

Plethysmography is measurement of volume, and changes in volume in the legs correlate with changes in venous pressure. Several systems are available, and they are all non-invasive and painless. Foot volume plethysmography works on the principle of an open water bath continuously measuring volume by displacement. Air plethysmography measures changes in calf volume, and strain gauge plethysmography measures limb circumference (and thereby volume) by assuming the limb to be a cylinder. In photoplethysmography a small transducer is used that consists of a diode that emits infrared light into the tissues with an adjacent photodetector that receives reflected light. This transducer is fixed to the patient's foot and the output signal is amplified and recorded. A shift from the baseline measurements represents a change in blood volume, which is in turn governed by venous pressure. This assessment is largely qualitative, though the other types of plethysmography are both easily standardised and quantitative.

All these measurements are used to assess the calf muscle pump by exercise testing as described for the venous pressure studies. In normal subjects exercise reduces the volume in the foot and calf as blood is expelled, and this returns to normal within 30-40 seconds of stopping exercise. Abnormal results in patients with deep venous obstruction or deep venous insufficiency are interpreted in exactly the same way as the direct pressure measurements.

In each of these quantitative tests the crucial question is whether the calf pump function returns to normal when the superficial veins are occluded by

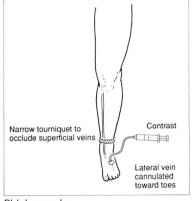

Phlebography.

a tourniquet. If it does, then the deep veins are normal. If not, the position of the tourniquet gives information about site of incompetence.

Phlebography

Ascending phlebography remains the most reliable test of deep venous anatomy. Similar techniques may be used in the diagnosis of chronic venous occlusion and will also show the extent of any collateral circulation.

Descending phlebography is used specifically to assess valvular incompetence. Under local infiltration anaesthesia the common femoral vein is cannulated at the groin and contrast medium injected while the patient carries out a Valsalva manoeuvre with the examination table tilted at 60° foot downwards. *x* Ray films are taken to determine how far down the leg the contrast medium has passed, and the results are graded on an arbitrary scale.

Lipodermatosclerosis and ulceration

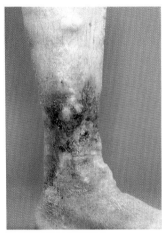

Calf perforating veins, lipodermatosclerosis, and early ulceration.

The incidence of lipodermatosclerosis and ulceration in patients who have had deep vein thromboses increases with time. The interval between the original thrombosis and the development of the postphlebitic syndrome may be 10-15 years, and probably depends on the tissue response to the venous hypertension. The actual changes in the venous circulation (either recanalisation or the development of a collateral circulation) occur much earlier and compensation is usually complete within three years. Some symptoms may precede frank ulceration by a long time and may start to develop within three years. Within 5-10 years three quarters of patients who had moderate or severe thromboses will have started to get symptoms and these will be severe in up to 40% of cases. The ultimate incidence of ulceration is 4-7%.

It is not possible to correlate accurately the extent of the thrombosis and the incidence of symptoms. The extent of dysfunction of the calf muscle pump as measured by plethysmography, however, does correlate with the incidence of post-thrombotic symptoms. Patients with deep venous insufficiency are at greater risk of developing these complications than patients with deep vein obstruction alone. If the venous pressure after exercise is less than 45 mm Hg the risk of ulceration is negligible, but when it is more than 60 mm Hg the incidence rises to more than 50%.

Treatment

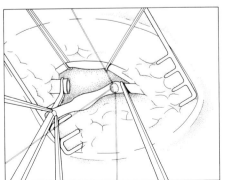

Support stockings reduce the risk of liposclerosis and ulceration.

Support stockings

Injury to a deep vein, whether it results in deep venous obstruction or deep venous insufficiency, requires lifelong treatment as soon as it is diagnosed if the postphlebitic syndrome is to be avoided. Patients should avoid prolonged periods of standing, and whenever they have the opportunity to sit the affected limb should be raised to encourage venous drainage.

Good quality fitted stockings that provide graduated compression (30-40 mm Hg) should be prescribed. Such stockings reduce the venous transmural pressure, improve the function of the calf muscle pump, and stimulate venous flow during recumbency, thereby reducing the risk of recurrent thrombosis.

Fibrinolytic enhancement

Although compression stockings reverse the skin changes of lipodermatosclerosis, some patients' condition may be further improved by the use of drugs which stimulate fibrinolysis, such as stanozolol.

Operation

Accurate assessment of calf pump function is essential before operation is contemplated. If calf pump dysfunction results from a combination of superficial varicose veins and incompetent perforating veins, then removal of varicose veins and ligation of perforating veins will repair the calf muscle pump and give good prospects for a long term cure. If the deep veins are incompetent the results of operation are poor, because the raised pressure in the deep veins rapidly leads to the re-emergence of incompetent communicating veins.

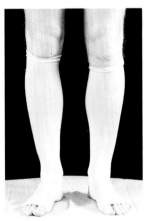

Replacement of incompetent femoral vein with valved segment from axilla.

Deep venous insufficiency and occlusion

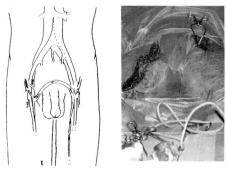

Diagram and operative photograph showing a Palma crossover vein bypass operation using the long saphenous vein from the normal leg (illustrating a left iliac vein occlusion).

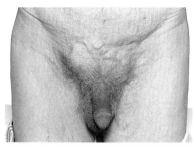

Many patients produce their own femorofemoral collaterals (note the suprapubic varicose veins). Operation in such patients is unnecessary.

There are no reliable and safe methods for repairing incompetent valves in deep veins. Research continues, however, and includes assessment of transplanting vein valves from the axillary vein into the upper popliteal segment. This has relieved symptoms in some patients, and calf pump function has been improved. Additional attempts have been made to repair femoral vein valves. This may have a place in patients with congenital valve aplasia, but so far there has been no long term follow up in patients who have undergone repair of valves after thrombosis in limbs. The support of incompetent valves with external slings has also been tried, with encouraging initial results.

Longstanding venous occlusion may be treated by bypass. The contralateral normal long saphenous vein is dissected out and anastomosed to the femoral vein on the occluded side. The iliac occlusion is bypassed and encouraging results have been obtained. The adjunctive use of a temporary arteriovenous fistula increases flow, and this maintains patency. Bypass of an occluded superficial femoral vein (using long saphenous vein) does not give equally good results.

Synthetic materials are rarely used in the venous system except as simple patches, but externally reinforced polytetrafluoroethylene is the material of choice for replacement of the iliac veins and the inferior vena cava.

VARICOSE VEINS

John T Hobbs

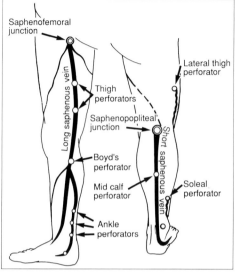

Clinically important veins of the leg: medial view (left) and posterolateral view (right).

Over 50 000 patients are admitted to British hospitals for treatment of varicose veins or their complications each year. Varicose veins cause much morbidity and their incidence is increasing, probably because of the modern Western diet and sedentary lifestyle. "Varicose" veins are dilated, lengthened, and tortuous superficial veins. Although they are sometimes thought of as "vanity" veins, the term "chronic venous insufficiency" gives a more accurate sense of the clinical problem.

In the United Kingdom two thirds of the adult population may show a venous problem at some time, and each year roughly half a million people (the female to male ratio is 5:1) consult their general practitioners about varicose veins. Because venous disease is seldom acute or life threatening these disorders have a low priority and are usually seen and treated by the least experienced member of the surgical team, often without supervision.

In addition to relief of symptoms and prevention of complications, the cosmetic aspects are important; women seek advice because of disfigurement and also because of complications they see in older people. Treatment is often inadequate or incorrect. If venous problems are carefully assessed and treated the symptoms can be relieved, in most cases with good long term results.

Presentation and aetiology

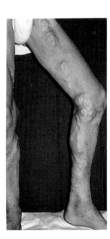

Atypical secondary veins with Klippel Trenaunay syndrome. Note obvious and distended lateral vein.

Primary varicose veins affecting the long saphenous system.

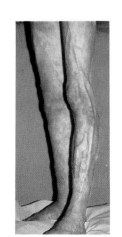

Types of vein

Athletic veins—Normal veins that are prominent on healthy muscular legs in non-obese people.

Dilated venules (also known as thread veins and spider bursts). These are the result of hormonal effects on soft skin and appear at the menarche, during pregnancy, with the menopause, and at other times of hormonal disturbance.

Primary varicose veins—These are often familial and caused by valvulvar incompetence and weakness of the vein wall.

Secondary varicose veins—These usually follow deep vein thrombosis as the post-thrombotic syndrome. More rarely they are a manifestation of arteriovenous shunting, usually the Klippel-Trenaunay syndrome but occasionally occurring as a result of trauma by gunshot, stab, or surgery.

Anatomy

The blood supply to the legs is considerable to meet the demands of active muscles and large bones, and this blood must be returned to the heart through the veins against gravity. The venous system of the legs comprises a superficial system in the skin and subcutaneous fat, and a deep system beneath the fascia. The superficial system is a venous network with prominent long and short saphenous veins, and these and other perforating veins pass through the deep fascia to join the deep veins. The superficial veins, the perforating veins, and the deep veins contain valves to prevent backflow.

51

Varicose veins

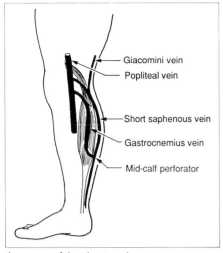

Anatomy of the short saphenous system.

Giacomini vein
Popliteal vein
Short saphenous vein
Gastrocnemius vein
Mid-calf perforator

Signs, symptoms, and complications of chronic venous insufficiency

- Unsightly varicose veins
- Tired, aching, heavy legs
- Ankle swelling
- Night cramps
- Restless legs
- Superficial thrombophlebitis
- Haemorrhage
- Irritation and venous eczema
- Lipodermatosclerosis
- Venous ulceration

Investigations

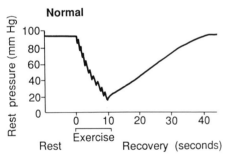

Normal

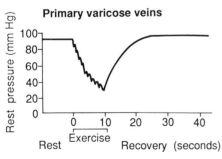

Primary varicose veins

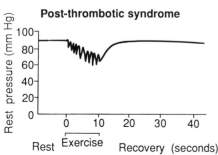

Post-thrombotic syndrome

Physiology

Blood is returned from the periphery by the pumping action of the muscles, which compress the deep veins that contain one way valves, and this is aided by the respiratory movements of the diaphragm. The chief muscular pumps are the muscles of the calf and foot. When deep veins are emptied, reflux is prevented by the valves and blood is sucked in from the superficial veins. When standing the pressure at the ankle is about 90 mm Hg, the height of a column of blood up to the heart. Muscular contractions of the calf reduce this pressure stepwise to a low plateau — known as the ambulatory venous pressure. At rest after exercise the pressure rises to the level before exercise.

In patients with primary varicose veins the drop in pressure is the same as in a normal leg, but the refilling time is much shorter. In patients with secondary varicose veins the pressure drop is much less than normal and is related to the severity of the venous damage.

Dilatation of superficial veins results in cosmetic disfigurement and occasional irritation. The most common symptoms are tiredness with aching, throbbing, "heavy" legs. They are worse when standing, in hot weather, before menstruation, and are relieved by walking. As soon as muscle activity ceases, however, the pressure rapidly rises again and the symptoms return.

Incompetence of the venous valves permits reflux and so the veins dilate and the pressure patterns become abnormal. The veins then become tortuous and varicose. Pregnant women are particularly prone to developing varicose veins because of the changes in blood hormone concentrations cause the vein walls to relax and dilate during the early stages of pregnancy, and later this dilatation is aggravated by the high pelvic blood flow. Additional factors are the retention of fluid and increased blood volume. Finally, there is considerable compression due to the enlarged uterus.

Many vascular laboratories have been established, and after initially being interested in arterial disease, they are now routinely investigating the venous system.

Measuring venous pressure is the most reliable way of studying venous haemodynamics but it is invasive. Many non-invasive methods have been introduced, including thermography, isotope phlebography, impedance plethysmography, air plethysmography, foot volumetry, photoplethysmography, light reflection rheography, Doppler ultrasonography, B mode ultrasonography, and, most recently, colour flow imaging. At present the best guide is a careful history and physical examination (including the use of a simple Doppler probe) combined with special investigations if these are inconclusive. The sites of incompetent perforating veins are best visualised by peroperative varicography.

The graphs show measurements of venous pressure in a normal leg, a leg with primary varicose veins, and a leg with the post-thrombotic syndrome. The exercise consisted of 10 tiptoe movements. The curves illustrate the fall in pressure in the normal leg and in primary varicose veins, but in the normal leg the recovery time is much longer. Because of the deep valvular incompetence in the post-thrombotic syndrome the drop in pressure is small and the recovery time short.

Treatment

Management of varicose veins

- Reassurance—including camouflage
- Support—elastic stockings
- Sclerotherapy
- Operation

Aide memoire for prescribing stockings

Q—**Quantity**: number of items
A—**Article**: type of stocking (drug tariff only "below knee" or "thigh" length; European Commission allows much greater range)
C—**Compression**: compression class I— 14-17 mm Hg; class II—18-24 mm Hg; class III—25-35 mm Hg; class IV—>35 mm Hg is available only from hospitals

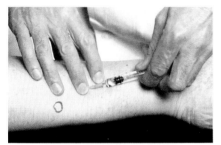

Marking of calf varicosities and injection of sclerosant.

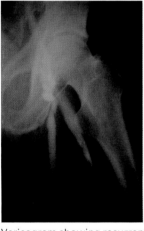

Varicogram showing recurrence at saphenofemoral junction (the needle marks previous incision).

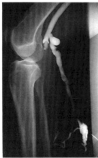

Varicogram showing saphenopopliteal junction with varix.

Not all leg symptoms are due to varicose veins, and some patients referred because of varicose veins do not require treatment for these as the real problem is an orthopaedic or arterial disorder.

During pregnancy, treatment should be conservative with appropriate but cosmetically acceptable support tights. If there is gross incompetence of the saphenofemoral junction causing much pain in the leg or vulval area, or an associated superficial thrombophlebitis, the saphenofemoral junction can be safely and simply divided under local anaesthesia, with immediate relief of symptoms.

Hosiery

Elastic stockings relieve symptoms, conceal veins, and prevent deterioration, but are not curative. Strong compression on the lower leg is required to prevent complications and should be graduated from the ankle, where problems are most common.

Types available range from those designed mainly for comfort and support to high strength (40 mm Hg) medical stockings for control of the disabling post-thrombotic syndrome, and for compression after treatment by injection.

Methods of measuring the pressure exerted by stockings are now available and a British Standards Institution Committee (BS 6612.85) has recommended that the pressure must be graduated. The recommended gradients are that the calf pressure should not be more than 75% of the pressure exerted at the ankle and the thigh pressure not more than 50%. The publication of this standard prompted the Department of Health to review the "elastic hosiery" section of the *Drug Tariff*. The aim of the new tariff is to draw attention to the performance of the stockings, and to clarify and simplify prescription.

Sclerotherapy

Veins can be eliminated either by sclerotherapy or operation and the two methods are complementary. Now that safe sclerosants are available all veins could be treated by injection if compression bandages could be applied and maintained for sufficient time. The aim of injection treatment is to place a small volume of an effective sclerosant in the lumen of the vein, which is then compressed to prevent formation of thrombus (clot). The compression must be maintained until permanent fibrosis has obliterated the lumen. After the initial period when the leg is bandaged, elastic stockings are worn daily until all tenderness, lumps, and discolouration have disappeared.

For large veins a 3% solution of sodium tetradecyl sulphate is most effective but may cause damage if used for small veins. Laser treatment of dilated venules has been abandoned because of poor results. Venules can be effectively and safely treated by injection, which is best done in a specialist clinic. Although complications are rare, the doctor must always be vigilant as there is a small risk of anaphylaxis. Resuscitation equipment must therefore always be immediately available.

Surgery

If there is proximal incompetence either in the groin or at the back of the knee operation is the only effective treatment because sclerotherapy rarely gives long lasting successful results at these sites.

Although general (or occasionally epidural) anaesthesia is used, patients are admitted on the day of operation and discharged home the following morning. Simple problems may be dealt with as day cases. The day after operation the bandages are removed and the small incisions covered with strips of permeable non-woven surgical synthetic adhesive tape. Medium strength elastic stockings are then worn during the day for a week until the stitches are removed. The stockings are removed at night for bathing and are left off overnight. Any residual veins can be dealt with by sclerotherapy.

Varicose veins

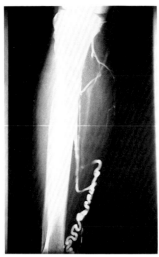

Varicogram showing
perforating vein of the lower leg.

Complications

Superficial thrombophlebitis is often confused with the potentially more dangerous deep vein thrombosis and treated with bed rest and potent anticoagulants. A firm bandage and instructions to walk are all that are required. Because of the signs of inflammation antibiotics are often prescribed, though bacterial infection never occurs in superficial thrombophlebitis. If there is an intravascular clot it should be evacuated by stabbing with a No 11 scalpel blade after applying a blob of local anaesthetic. Rarely the phlebitis spreads proximally to the groin and if seen within the first week may be dealt with by simple operation. This requires only an overnight admission, gives immediate relief, and is a means of long term cure; the pain of operation is less in both extent and duration than the pain that occurs when the condition is treated conservatively.

Venous ulcers are often treated as they were during the previous century but with the additional use of expensive local dressings which are not necessary and may even aggravate the condition. Patients are sometimes seen and treated by district nurses, often without supervision from the general practitioner or hospital consultant. Venous ulcers are fully discussed in the article on leg ulcers.

Conclusions

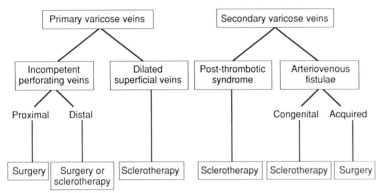

Management of varicose veins.

Because venous problems are so common and cause much long term morbidity they should be treated in special vein clinics because the more acute and potentially lethal conditions rightly take precedence in general and arterial surgical clinics. The vein clinics should be staffed by doctors who are equally enthusiastic and competent in both sclerotherapy and surgical treatment and are familiar with the problems. Consistently good results can be obtained if treatment is precisely planned and properly executed.

LEG ULCERS

E L Gilliland, John H N Wolfe

Ulceration of the lower leg is a common symptom that will affect 2% of people in their lifetime. Its prevalence increases with age from 0·5% among patients over 40 to 2% among those over 80. As the proportion of elderly people in the population increases, therefore, we can expect a rise in the present estimated numbers of leg ulcers unless a more educated approach to their management is taken.

Although some patients tolerate their ulcers, to others the condition is smelly and painful, resulting in time off work (500 000 working days/year), perhaps loss of a job, social isolation, and—in a few cases—complete disability. Though important advances have been made in the management of many chronic conditions, the management of leg ulcers in some parts of the United Kingdom lags far behind the standards set by some European countries. Treatment is fragmented, poorly taught, and inadequately researched; the average time taken to heal an ulcer is about six months; and some persist for years.

The present annual expenditure on the treatment of ulcers in the United Kingdom is about £50m—a large market for new products for ulcer care. Good management, however, depends on accurate diagnosis, simple and appropriate care of the wound, and treatment of the underlying cause.

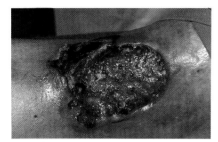

Extensive ulcer of lower leg with necrosis and granulation tissue.

Diagnosis

95% of leg ulcers are vascular, other causes are:

Neuropathy:	Haematological:
Diabetes	Sickle cell disease
Alcohol	Miscellaneous:
Infection	Pyoderma
Trauma	gangrenosum
Cancer (squamous)	Pressure sores

Rare causes of leg ulcers

Arteriovenous	Kaposi's sarcoma
malformation	Haemolytic jaundice
Syringomyelia	Leukaemia
Syphilis	Factitious causes
Basal cell cancer	Drugs
Melanoma	

Estimated number of leg ulcers treated each year

	District of 200 000 people	United Kingdom
Venous	200	63 000
Arterial (large vessel)	30	9 000
Arterial (small vessel)	15	4 500
Venous/arterial	30	9 000

A detailed history is essential because although most ulcers are caused by venous disease, other common causes—arteriosclerosis of main vessels, neuropathy, and disease of the small arteries—must not be missed. A venous ulcer is easily recognised when it is situated in the "gaiter" region near the medial malleolus, and occasionally adjacent to the lateral malleolus; it has a shallow base with a flat margin and the surrounding skin has features of long standing venous hypertension—haemosiderin pigmentation, atrophie blanche, eczema, and dilated venules over the instep of the foot (lipodermatosclerosis). In some cases ulcers may become circumferential.

Ischaemic ulcers can occur anywhere below the knee, but are most commonly seen on the foot and they are more likely to be painful than venous ulcers. The diagnosis may be difficult as—particularly in elderly people—there may be no history of claudication. These ulcers are often deep and invade deep fascia, tendon, and bone; associated local signs include pallor, dependent redness, dystrophic nails, reduced skin temperature, sluggish venous filling, and poor capillary return.

When arterial insufficiency is suspected or when oedema and local induration do not permit confident assessment of peripheral circulation, it is simple to auscultate the arteries with a portable Doppler probe and—with a sphygmomanometer placed around the calf—measure the systolic pressure in each of the three ankle vessels (peroneal, anterior tibial, and posterior tibial). The ratio of ankle:brachial pressure is a guide to the severity of the arterial disease. The routine use of Doppler ultrasound has shown that at least 10% of venous ulcers are accompanied by unrecognised arterial disease and it is these patients who are easy to mismanage. Any ulcer

Leg ulcers

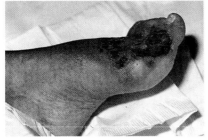

Ulcer resulting from small vessel arteritis.

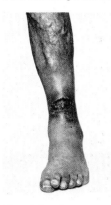

Ulcer following trauma in a patient with peripheral neuropathy.

Principles of management:
- Define the cause
- Treat the ulcer carefully
- Treat the underlying cause

with associated arterial disease should be referred to a vascular surgeon as inappropriate compression may cause irreversible tissue damage that will require amputation of the limb.

When foot pulses are easily palpable, appreciable atherosclerotic obstruction of the large vessels is unlikely so disease of the small vessels associated with diabetes, rheumatoid arthritis, and autoimmune diseases must be considered, particularly if multiple "punched out" ulcers are present. Thrombocythaemia and polycythaemia may also lead to ulceration and when venous disease is also present the diagnosis is easily missed. Until the underlying disease is treated or goes into remission the "venous" ulcer may remain unhealed despite otherwise adequate local treatment.

Skin cancers comprise up to 2% of ulcers seen in specialist clinics and are easy to misdiagnose unless the possibility of malignancy is kept in mind and a biopsy specimen taken. Features that suggest such a diagnosis include unusual or overabundant granulation tissue and rolled irregular edges; these may be either presenting features or they may develop in an ulcer that has remained unhealed for many years and undergone malignant change (Marjolin's ulcer). Early referral of patients with atypical ulcers, or ones that will not heal, will avoid inappropriate treatment.

Before outlining the treatment of leg ulcers we must emphasise that their prevention is of primary importance; patients with vascular disease or neuropathy affecting the legs have an increased risk of ulceration and should be advised and treated accordingly. Only a small proportion of patients with venous insufficiency will ever develop an ulcer even if deep venous insufficiency is present. Skin changes—in particular lipodermatosclerosis—around the malleoli should alert the practitioner to advise the patient to avoid local trauma, and complications such as eczema or ulceration require prompt treatment. Below knee stockings should be worn all day, and patients with arteriopathy or neuropathy, or both (especially diabetic patients), should be given advice about footwear and foot care and—if necessary—be referred to a chiropodist with a special interest in such problems.

Treatment

Factors impairing wound healing

Local:	General:
Reduced blood supply	Age
	Anaemia
Infection	Steroids
Mechanical stress	Diabetes
Denervation	Uraemia
Iatrogenic	Malnutrition
Presence of tumour	Vitamin deficiency
	Zinc deficiency
	Ambient temperature

There is no universally correct way to treat an ulcer as each patient's age, general health, social circumstances, and physical state must be taken into account. Anyone treating leg ulcers, however, from district nurse to consultant, must always be aware that there are two aspects of treatment—to promote healing by second intention and to treat the underlying cause. The decision about whether to treat patients in the community, refer them to a specialist clinic, or admit them to hospital must be based on local facilities and the response of the ulcer to initial treatment.

Local treatment to encourage healing by second intention

Soft tissue wounds heal by a complex process starting with granulation and progressing by migration of epithelium from the edges of the wound. Treatment of the systemic factors is self explanatory but the deleterious effects of steroids applied topically or given systemically, malnutrition (especially in elderly people), and the vasoconstrictive effects of a consistently low ambient temperature may be forgotten.

An ulcer may quickly become colonised by a wide variety of bacteria, so frequent cleansing with removal of slough and dead tissue is essential. Many products are promoted for their cleansing and healing effects with little or no clinical evidence to support their use. There is experimental evidence that certain commonly used cleansing agents (for example, eusol, chlorhexidine, and hydrogen peroxide) are toxic both to bacteria and to cells, and may therefore retard healing; others that contain lanolin (including all steroid ointments), hydroxybenzoates (Aserbine and

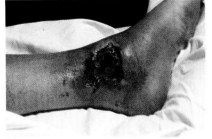

Extending infected ulcer with necrosis in a patient with pyoderma gangrenosum.

Antiseptics   Antibiotics

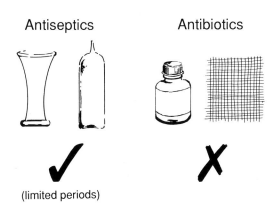

✓   ✗

(limited periods)

Preparations for local treatment

	No of preparations	
	Available	Recommended
Disinfectants/ cleansing agents	>30	Saline Povidone iodine Silver sulphadiazine Potassium permanganate
Dressings	>18	Paraffin gauze Sterile gauze
Medicated bandages		Cotton impregnated with zinc paste and hydroxybenzoates Cotton impregnated with icthammol and zinc oxide
Retention bandages	>12	Stretch fabric or tubular seamless gauze
Support stockings	>30	Medium/high compression (25-40 mm Hg)

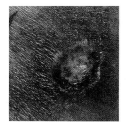

Stasis ulcer.

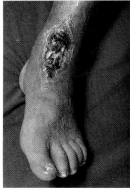

Deep ulcer with necrosis caused by tight bandaging of a leg with arterial disease.

Malatex), chlorocresol (Betnovate cream), colophony (Secaderm), and neomycin often cause sensitivity reactions that complicate the treatment.

Our advice is to debride dirty ulcers with a scalpel and forceps; when necessary a local anaesthetic can be applied topically or injected subcutaneously around the ulcer away from its edge. Eusol or hydrogen peroxide may be used instead of a scalpel but should be used only for limited periods; sterile saline or boiled tap water may then be used to wash the ulcer. Some particularly large or deep ulcers may require treatment in hospital by debridement under general anaesthesia.

Skin surrounding ulcers, particularly vascular ulcers, is rarely normal. Hyperkeratosis is common and usually the result of poor local hygiene or infrequent dressings. Excessive keratin harbours bacteria and may obscure other ulcers so it should be removed with tissue forceps; sometimes it is necessary to apply arachis oil or paraffin gauze for several days before attempting debridement. Patients should be encouraged to bathe with the leg wrapped in a polythene bag, or just before a visit by the district nurse so that the dressing can be soaked off. Peeling off an adherent dressing should be avoided as it may avulse granulation tissue and regenerating epithelium.

Antiseptics applied topically are acceptable, but antibiotics applied topically should be avoided. We recommend povidone iodine as the antiseptic for general use, silver sulphadiazine for short periods if *Pseudomonas* spp have been cultured, and potassium permanganate (1/8000 dilution) for wet ulcers with surrounding eczema—but again only for limited periods as it can cause local hyperkeratosis.

When cellulitis is present a swab of the ulcer must be taken before an antibiotic is prescribed; the most likely organism is *Staphylococcus aureus*. Further measures must include rest with elevation of the limb. Failure to respond to treatment, increasing cellulitis, or rapid enlargement of the ulcer, warrant immediate referral to hospital for treatment with systemic antibiotics.

What about non-adherent dressings and occlusive dressings? There is no such thing as a non-adherent dressing but paraffin gauze cut to the shape of the ulcer, three to four layers thick, is cheap and better than all the others. Occlusive dressings may offer some advantages but they can aggravate local infection and their place in the management of ulcers has yet to be established. Skin is the best dressing and can be applied either as a partial thickness graft or as numerous pinch grafts. It is best reserved for large ulcers or those that will not heal by conservative treatment, and success rates of up to 90% can be achieved by selecting cases carefully, cleaning the ulcers, careful follow up, and treating the underlying cause.

Treating the cause

As with any other medical problem treatment is often a compromise between what should be done, what can be done, and what the patient wants to be done. General advice on weight loss, regular exercise, and ankle exercises to improve venous return should be given, together with a simple explanation of the rationale of the treatment to improve compliance.

Adequate graduated compression is sufficient to heal most venous ulcers; below knee compression stockings that exert a pressure of at least 20-25 mm Hg at the ankle are most suitable and should heal 80-90% of venous ulcers that are <10 cm^2 within three months. Unfortunately the stockings that provide this degree of compression (Venosan 2002, Sigvaris 504, Jobst, and Medi) are not available except on prescription in hospitals.

The two main drawbacks to high grade compression stockings—discomfort and difficulty in application—may be overcome by simple modifications in policy. If high grade compression is unbearable, then TED stockings, two layers of Tubigrip, or a well padded paste bandage—though they give less compression—may still heal the ulcer, after which compression can be increased. Elderly or infirm patients who cannot apply the stockings should wear them continuously and the district nurse or a relative may change them twice a week. Advice on other measures to control oedema is equally important—never stand when you can sit, never sit when you can lie down (preferably with the legs above the level of the chest), and put blocks under the foot of the bed or sleep with the legs on a pillow, or both. When ankle movements are restricted, simple exercises, physiotherapy, and regular attention to gait should improve the function of the calf muscles and the venous return.

Leg ulcers

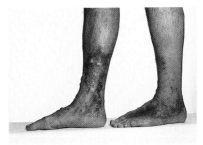

Stasis ulcer with eczema and pigmentation.

Ischaemic ulcers require a different approach as they may lead to irreversible ischaemia and amputation. A vascular surgeon's opinion should be sought early even for elderly patients as major reconstructive surgery, percutaneous transluminal angioplasty, or a chemical (phenol) sympathectomy may be beneficial. The presence of both venous and arterial disease in an ulcerated leg complicates management as their relative contributions to the pathophysiology are difficult to define even after extensive investigations. On the one hand graded compression may aggravate local ischaemia, and on the other hand improved arterial inflow may aggravate the venous insufficiency.

A manageable balance by the year 2000?

Estimate of possible savings

Assuming:

- It takes one hour/week to dress each ulcer
- It costs £10/week to dress each ulcer
- Average time to healing is six months

Then:

- Healing time of 100 ulcers can be reduced by two months
- The total number of ulcers is reduced by 50 after a year

So:

- Savings = Dressings   £22 000
  Nursing time   £10 000

Failure to heal a leg ulcer is usually the result of poor clinical acumen or inappropriate care of the wound; the blame rarely lies with the patient, though there are a few patients whose comprehension and motivation will never permit more than temporary success. With increasing numbers of people living to be over the age of 80 the incidence of leg ulcers may double by the year 2000, so unless a concerted effort is made to improve treatment and prevent recurrence resources will have to be increased or patients will suffer. New and more expensive dressings are not the answer until we assess critically the results of our present treatments.

The number of leg ulcers in a community can be reduced by a combination of active management, a simple and unified policy of treatment within a district with nurses specifically appointed to manage leg ulcers, and a specialist clinic for the assessment of the intractable, painful, and large ulcers. Improvements in healing time with a reduction in total numbers could achieve substantial savings within one or two years. With a more unified approach proper clinical trials of specific problems could further improve ulcer care with consequent savings of time and money.

THE SWOLLEN LEG

D T Reilly, John H N Wolfe

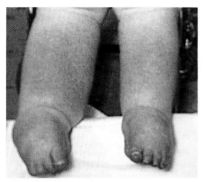

Dependent oedema in a patient with poliomyelitis.

In both hospital and general practice the patient with a swollen leg presents a common dilemma in diagnosis and treatment. The cause may be trivial or life threatening—an insect bite or a deep vein thrombosis—and it is difficult to negotiate the path between overinvestigation and laissez faire.
Fortunately in most cases the decision becomes clear after a careful history has been taken and a clinical examination carried out.

Pathophysiology

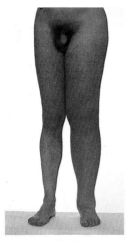
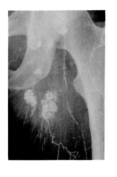

Pelvic lymphatic obstruction shown clinically (left) and radiographically (right) with a profusion of abnormal lymphatics running into inguinal lymph nodes but no lymphatics running into the pelvis.

It is helpful to return to simple physiological concepts to understand the development of swelling of the lower limb. In a normal limb the hydrostatic pressure of the column of blood in the veins is balanced by the calf muscle pump, which depends for its efficiency on the integrity of the venous valves as well as on the ability of the muscle to contract. Thus several causes of swelling are immediately apparent: postphlebitic damage to valves, prolonged dependency (as in a leg with rest pain), or failure of the muscle pump (as in a paralysed limb or an arthritic limb with fixity of the ankle joint). The period of rest and elevation of the limb every night normally permits resolution of any slight oedema that may have built up during the day: if this normal behaviour is prevented (as during a prolonged flight) oedema results.

The redistribution of fluid from the arterial end of the capillary to the venous end (Starling's law) explains the mechanisms of the production of oedema. Venous hypertension causes increased pressure in the postcapillary venule and thus back diffusion of fluid into the tissues; lower plasma oncotic pressure also prevents tissue fluid returning to the vein from the interstitial space. Increased capillary permeability (accompanying injury or allergy) will cause oedema by exudation of fluid rich in protein into the tissue spaces. Failure to remove protein—and therefore fluid—because of lymphatic insufficiency is the other main cause of oedema.

Clinical features

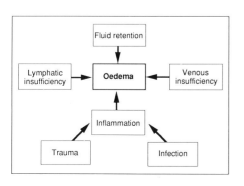

Causes of both acute and chronic swelling of the leg can be grouped into:
- *General*—fluid retention as in cardiac and renal failure, and hypoproteinaemia
- *Local*—venous or lymphatic insufficiency
- *Inflammatory*—allergy, trauma, or infection.

Much can be gained from examination of the affected limb, particularly the pattern of the swelling: if the oedema is maximal in the ankles and legs, and the feet are spared, the cause is more likely to be venous than lymphatic.

The swollen leg

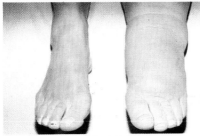

Lymphoedema of the left foot (note the square toes).

Deposition of haemosiderin and atrophic or ulcerated skin also favour a venous cause, whereas diffuse long standing oedema that is most prominent distally with hypertrophied lichenified skin is the picture of lymphoedema. It is often stated that cardiac oedema pits and lymphatic oedema does not, but all oedema pits initially and becomes brawny as fibrin is deposited in the intercellular spaces. We will consider here only local causes, assuming that systemic causes have been excluded.

The acutely swollen leg

Local causes

- Trauma
- Deep vein thrombosis
- Allergy
- Cellulitis
- Snake or insect bite
- Rheumatological disease

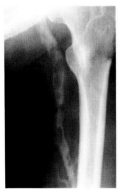

Venogram showing deep vein thrombosis.

Trauma and allergy, insect bite and cellulitis, can rapidly be differentiated. Examination should show a portal of entry and should also pick up such traumatic causes as undisplaced fracture (bony tenderness) or haematoma (bruising and fluctuance). Rheumatological causes should be suspected if there is a joint effusion or a skin rash (for example, erythema nodosum), and a ruptured Baker's cyst is usually easy to feel. Lymphoedema is painless unless there is associated cellulitis.

The cause that cannot confidently be diagnosed or excluded on clinical grounds is the most worrying—that is, deep vein thrombosis. It is still sometimes asserted that clinical signs are enough, and consequently some patients without deep vein thrombosis receive long term anticoagulant treatment because of a confident clinical diagnosis. Sufficient studies have now been carried out to show that 20-30% of the patients with signs and symptoms will fail to show a deep vein thrombosis on venography. Conversely, exclusion of deep vein thrombosis by clinical examination alone is wrong half the time. Characteristically an acute deep vein thrombosis (if it causes clinical signs) produces tense swelling of the deep compartment and not just superficial oedema. Management of deep vein thrombosis is discussed in the article on thrombosis and pulmonary embolism.

The chronically swollen leg

Local causes

- Venous:
  Postphlebitic limb
  Venous compression
  Varicose veins
- Lymphoedema:
  Primary
  Secondary
- Congenital malformation
- Dependency

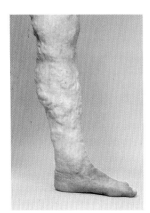

Swelling caused by venous disease.

The mainstay of treatment of patients with chronically swollen legs (once systemic causes have been excluded) is compression with elastic stockings, so it may be argued that there is little point in investigation if the treatment is to be the same. This is a counsel of despair: there are a number of surgical options available for a subgroup of patients with venous or lymphatic insufficiency, and this minority will be denied adequate treatment if the right diagnosis is never made. Prognosis depends on diagnosis—for instance, the patient with lymphoedema will be advised to have immediate treatment with antibiotics for minor infections of the affected limb to prevent loss by fibrosis of further scarce lymph vessels.

History and examination

The common causes of chronic swelling are venous and lymphatic insufficiency; several other causes can, however, be diagnosed on clinical grounds alone. For example, a common source of confusion is arterial insufficiency; a patient immobilised with rest pain may sleep in a chair or leave his or her foot dangling over the side of the bed, so that the most obvious feature is oedema of the foot and leg. Here the history and pain in the calf on dorsiflexion of the foot are usually enough to make the diagnosis. Similarly, the immobility of a patient with a cerebrovascular accident may lead to oedema in the affected leg that may simulate a deep vein thrombosis.

Venous causes—A history of deep vein thrombosis should always be sought, but will often be non-existent even in the presence of the typical appearance of the leg with chronic venous insufficiency—that is, a swollen, brawny, pigmented calf with eczema or ulcers. There may be obvious varicose veins. Occasionally primary varicose veins can be the cause of swelling and ulceration, but usually varicose veins in a patient with these

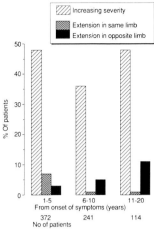

Progress of lymphoedema.

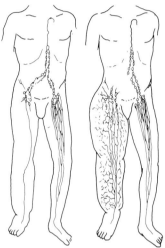

Distal lymphatic obliteration (left) and pelvic obstruction (right). Distal obliteration occurs almost exclusively in women, and is mild. Pelvic obstruction occurs in twice as many women as men, and is severe.

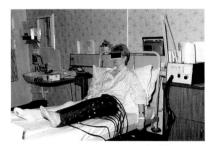

Lymphoedema being treated with a Lymphapress.

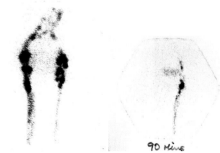

Normal isotope lymphogram (left) and distal obliteration with no clearance in the right leg (right).

chronic changes are incidental to deep venous obstruction or damage to the valves that is causing reflux. In the absence of postphlebitic changes—for example, in the aching fat leg—the presence of minor varicosities is unlikely to be of importance. Muscular cramps and aching legs are occasionally symptoms of venous insufficiency but are unreliable. If venous claudication is really present, a history of a progressively worsening "bursting" pain on walking will be elicited.

The appropriate patients to refer for investigation of suspected chronic venous problems are those with obvious varicose veins, those with venous claudication, and—in particular—working people whose lives are made difficult by swelling, pain, or ulcers. Obese patients and those who have other problems such as cardiac failure and who spend most of their time immobile in a chair generally do not respond to treatment. In the vascular laboratory a range of investigations is available. The most useful of these are venous Doppler studies, venous pressure measurement, plethysmography, and duplex ultrasound scanning. These investigations can exclude a venous cause for the patient's problem or add functional information (such as the presence or absence of deep or superficial reflux or deep vein obstruction) and the newer duplex Doppler imaging system can show venous architecture and valve function.

The purpose of the investigations is to identify the subgroup of patients who will benefit from operations. The operations range from high ligation, stripping, and avulsion of varicose veins and subfascial ligation of perforators to the more complex operations for deep obstruction or reflux for which bypass grafting or vein and valve transplantation may be possible. Vein and valve transplantation is still being evaluated.

Most chronic venous problems are not amenable to surgical correction and conservative treatment is centred on adequate compression with specially fitted stockings, which need to be renewed roughly every six months. Below knee stockings are usually sufficient; full length stockings tend to roll down and "ruck" behind the knee.

Lymphatic causes—The huge "elephantiasis" leg of severe long standing lymphatic obstruction is obvious, but most patients present with unilateral painless oedema in a healthy looking leg with no features of venous insufficiency. These patients fall into four major categories. Most are young women with mild oedema and their prognosis is good; the oedema is unlikely to progress to the thigh and adequate conservative treatment should suffice (category 1). There is a group, however, who present with a more aggressive onset of oedema affecting both calf and thigh; these patients are likely to have patent distal lymphatics but ilioinguinal obstruction, and are the group who may benefit from early investigation with a view to mesenteric bridge lymphatic bypass. Good results are possible if this is done before obliteration of the distal lymphatics has occurred (category 2). A few may have an associated capillary naevus; this is indicative of megalymphatics that may also respond to surgical intervention (category 3). Cutaneous lymph or chylous vesicles are a sign of lymphatic reflux, and patients who have these incompetent refluxing lymphatics may have associated chylous ascites, chylothorax, or—more rarely—chylometrorrhoea, chyluria, or malabsorption. Ligation of the relevant lymphatics can produce immediate relief of symptoms (category 4).

The diagnosis of lymphoedema is often a diagnosis of exclusion except in a severe case. The indications for further investigation of the lymphatic system are: (*a*) when the diagnosis is in doubt, and (*b*) if ilioinguinal obstruction is suspected. Investigation is usually by a colloid labelled with a radioisotope.

Radionuclide lymphography uses high energy emitters bound to colloids which are taken up by the lymphatic vessels; it has the advantages of safety and a lower dose of radiation, and there is the opportunity to do studies of clearance rates, which may provide useful functional information.

For bipedal lymphography the lymphatic vessels in the dorsum of the foot have firstly to be identified by injection of a diffusible dye into the web space, and then dissected out and cannulated under magnification. Radio-opaque ethiodised oil (Lipiodol) is then injected and its progress followed radiologically. This is time consuming, and there is always the danger of pulmonary or cerebral oil embolism. If it is impossible to find peripheral lymphatic vessels to cannulate, the diagnosis of distal obliteration is confirmed. Megalymphatics or inguinal obstruction may also be seen.

The swollen leg

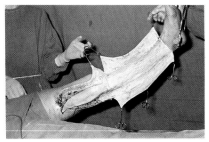

Homan's operation for lymphoedema.

Treatment of lymphoedema

For 90% of cases

- Use of grade IV elastic support stocking
- Raising the foot of the bed at night
- Use of pneumatic compression pump and legging
- Use of antiseptic soap and foot hygiene to prevent infection and cellulitis in feet

For 10% of cases

- Excision of lymphoedematous subcutaneous fat (for gross lymphoedema)
- Ligation of lymphatic fistula (for megalymphatics)
- Ileal mesenteric bridging (for pelvic obstruction)

It is not usually possible to cure lymphoedema but an active and enthusiastic approach can achieve great benefit. Most patients require only conservative treatment but if this is rigorously applied the results can be good. A short period of treatment in hospital using a Lymphapress can alter the patient's perception of the leg and engender enthusiasm for self treatment; cellulitis must be avoided by rigorous attention to hygiene.

A few patients benefit from operation, but this must never be carried out for cosmetic reasons. Those with heavy cumbersome legs can have the volume of subcutaneous tissue removed (Homan's operation) and the results are usually good if the indications for operation are correct. Such operations may also permit support hosiery to fit better.

A small group may benefit from operations to relieve lymphatic obstruction (mesenteric ileal bridging operation or direct lymphovenous anastomosis) but this group does not impinge on the mass of patients who should be treated conservatively.

The diagrams of distal obliteration and pelvic obstruction are reproduced by permission of the publisher, Butterworth Heinemann, from DeWeese J, ed. Vascular surgery. In: Dudley H, Carter D, eds. *Rob and Smith's operative surgery.* 4th ed. 1985, 361.

CAROTID ENDARTERECTOMY

D J Thomas, John H N Wolfe

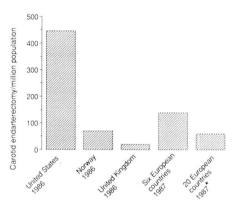

Number of carotid endarterectomies carried out/million population, 1986-7.
*(Information obtained from questionnaire sent to surgeons.)

Current practice

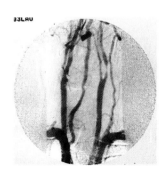

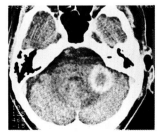

Angiogram of patient with vertebrobasilar symptoms and a 70% left internal carotid stenosis (top). Computed tomogram (bottom) showed secondary deposit in the cerebellum from an occult primary growth in the bronchus.

Carotid endarterectomy has been done for 35 years. Patients who have experienced transient visual loss or cerebral ischaemic attacks may have the operation as prophylaxis against unilateral blindness or stroke. Transient ischaemic attacks often stop immediately, and the risk of stroke once the perioperative period is past may be as low as 1% a year. It has been the most common vascular operation in the United States, with roughly 100 000 such operations being done each year. About half of these operations were done for patients with asymptomatic carotid disease.

In the best hands perioperative morbidity or mortality are less than 3%, but many operations are not done in major vascular centres and perioperative complication rates of up to 15% have been quoted. The operation that is supposed to prevent stroke may actually be causing more than 10 000 strokes a year in the United States alone. A backlash has developed from insurance agencies and the government, and surgeons now have to justify each procedure.

Patients who present with transient ischaemic attacks are a heterogeneous group. In those with carotid stenosis the risks of angiography and surgery need to be balanced against the expected natural history for each patient. The interim results of two important trials have recently been published, which help to clarify the role of carotid endarterectomy in certain subgroups.

There has been an increasing tendency to treat these patients with aspirin and not to seek a specialist opinion at all, despite the fact that the protective effect of antiplatelet drugs is not impressive. The results of the carotid endarterectomy trials should change this approach.

In the United Kingdom, patients with probable transient ischaemic attacks and carotid stenosis are often referred directly to a vascular surgeon without first seeing a neurologist. This is analagous to a person with undiagnosed chest pain being referred directly to a cardiac surgeon without first being assessed by a physician or cardiologist. This practice is undesirable because many transient symptoms are not vascular in origin and some that are may not be relevant to a carotid stenosis. Many patients have symptoms caused by disease in the vertebrobasilar system, some patients have focal symptoms produced by migrainous phenomena, and others may have focal epilepsy—with or without a cerebral tumour.

Until relatively recently, accurate imaging of the carotid bifurcation sufficient to permit operation needed intra-arterial angiography. In high risk vascular patients, this is not without its risks. Possibly 3% of patients will have a transient neurological problem at the time of angiography and 1% may have some residual deficit. Fortunately, it is now possible to image the carotid bifurcation more safely. This can be done with Doppler ultrasonography, magnetic resonance angiography, or intravenous digital subtraction angiography. Clinicians are far less inhibited by these safe investigations and the number of carotid bifurcations imaged is likely to escalate. Once a stenosis has been seen it may be hard to ignore, but careful appraisal is necessary—merely finding a stenosis is not sufficient reason for operating on it.

If a patient is found to have chronic complete occlusion of the internal carotid artery then disobliteration is not possible.

Natural history

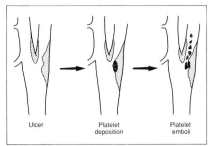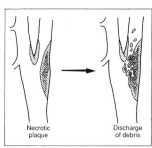

Two ways in which emboli develop from a carotid plaque: (left) a thrombus of platelet emboli form in an ulcerated plaque (which would presumably respond to treatment with aspirin); and (right) discharge of atheromatous debris from an ulcerating plaque (which is unlikely to respond to either anticoagulants or aspirin).

The natural history of patients presenting with transient ischaemic attacks is becoming clearer. When large numbers of such patients are grouped together, a stroke rate of 5-10% a year can be expected. The United Kingdom transient ischaemic attack aspirin trial of 2500 patients showed that for every 100 patients in the control group with such attacks followed up for two years, 14 had a stroke or myocardial infarction, or died of vascular disease. In patients taking aspirin the corresponding figure was 11. It should be emphasised that this difference was not significant. It was only when the results were combined with the results of several other studies of the effect of antiplatelet drugs that the difference achieved significance.

Patients presenting with transient monocular blindness alone, and having no other vascular risk factors, have a lower risk of stroke, possibly 1-2% a year. In contrast, patients with risk factors such as hypertension, ischaemic heart disease, peripheral vascular disease, and diabetes, may have a much higher annual risk rate than the 5-7% generally quoted.

Reliability of clinical signs

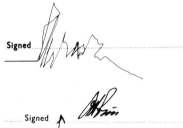

Signature before carotid endarterectomy carried out during crescendo transient ischaemic attacks (top) and after carotid endarterectomy (bottom).

A bruit over the carotid bifurcation is not necessarily caused by stenosis of the internal carotid artery. More importantly, the absence of a bruit does not exclude severe carotid disease. A bruit may be merely a flow murmur in patients with anaemia or thyrotoxicosis. It may be conducted up the carotid arteries from the aortic valve or from the innominate or subclavian arteries. In patients with disease of the carotid bifurcation it might be generated from the external carotid artery, and the internal carotid artery may be relatively free of atheroma or even completely occluded. When a stenosis exceeds 85% its bruit may disappear because flow rate through the stenosis starts to fall. It is not uncommon to find a bruit over the contralateral asymptomatic stenosis and no audible bruit on the symptomatic side. The presence of a bruit anywhere in the neck should therefore be taken as indicative of arterial stenosis in a patient at risk, and Doppler ultrasonography should be recommended for screening these patients.

Interim results of current trials

> **Present situations in two trials of carotid endarterectomy**
>
> - Both trials have stopped randomising patients with >70% stenosis
> - Both trials have shown that operation is better than medical treatment alone if stenosis is >70%, providing that the operative stroke rate is <6%
> - The European trial has shown that there is no place for operation if stenosis is <30%
> - There are not yet any clear answers for stenoses between 30% and 70%

Both the European and North American carotid trials have shown that patients with symptomatic carotid stenosis that exceeds 70% will benefit from carotid endarterectomy, provided it can be done with a perioperative complication rate of less than 6%. Surgery reduces the risk of ipsilateral stroke by almost 50% in patients with severe stenosis. This beneficial effect is not apparent during the early months because of the perioperative risk. The benefit starts to accrue after one year, so patients who have a poor general prognosis and are unlikely to live for 12 months because of other disease should not be offered operation.

The European study randomised patients with less than 30% stenosis. Carotid endarterectomy is not justified in this group since so few patients with this degree of stenosis go on to have ipsilateral stroke.

For patients with stenoses between 30% and 70% the effect remains to be clarified, and both studies are continuing to randomise patients in this group.

Asymptomatic stenoses

> **Unless there are overriding considerations, patients with symptomatic carotid stenosis of more than 70% should have a carotid endarterectomy**

The management of patients with asymptomatic carotid stenosis is not as straightforward as at first it may seem. There is a natural reluctance to advise operation on a patient with no symptoms. From monitoring patients for peripheral vascular disease who are known to have coincidental asymptomatic tight carotid stenosis, however, it is clear that some patients go on to have strokes.

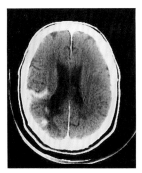

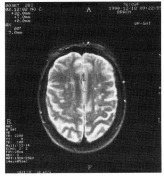

Angiogram showing severe bilateral carotid stenoses (top). These were asymptomatic, but the computed tomogram (bottom) showed evidence of bilateral cerebral infarction.

A large part of the brain gives no signs that a small ischaemic event has occurred, and some patients with no symptoms have been shown on computed tomography to have small infarcts. Magnetic resonance imaging, which is many times more sensitive than computed tomography in detecting vascular lesions, may show definite evidence of small infarcts in the hemisphere ipsilateral to a tight "asymptomatic carotid stenosis."

The beneficial results of treating patients with symptoms from tight carotid stenoses, and the acknowledgement that a patient who has been free of symptoms may have had small infarcts and may go on to develop a stroke, have encouraged the creation of multicentre trials of the effects of carotid endarterectomy in patients with no symptoms, and the results are eagerly awaited.

Patients with severe carotid stenoses are at risk from stroke if they undergo major operations—especially coronary artery bypass grafting—during which hypotension is likely. As yet there is no clear evidence that carotid endarterectomy for asymptomatic disease reduces the incidence of stroke after coronary artery bypass grafting. The trials to date have included rather small numbers of patients, however, and further investigation of this important issue is required.

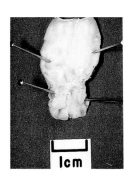 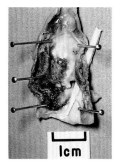

Two specimens from carotid endarterectomy that both showed as severe stenosis in the angiogram. One may be benign (left) with an ivory smooth plaque, and the other (right) is ulcerated and could be the source of emboli.

Indications for operation

> ## Indications for carotid endarterectomy
>
> - Tight (>70%) carotid stenosis giving symptoms
> - Failed medical treatment of a clinically appropriate carotid stenosis
> - Inability to take aspirin or anticoagulants for a clinically appropriate carotid stenosis
> - Thrombus visible in lumen on angiography
> - Flow distal to the stenosis so severely reduced that occlusion is likely to develop
>
> (Perioperative complication rate must be less than 6%)

Firstly, patients with symptomatic carotid disease and a stenosis exceeding 70% should be offered surgery. Secondly, patients should be considered who have an operable carotid stenosis and who despite taking antiplatelet or anticoagulant treatment continue to have transient ischaemic attacks. Thirdly, patients who are unable to take antiplatelet or anticoagulant drugs—for example, because of peptic ulceration—should also be considered. Caution should be exercised when referring patients for operation who have high risk features like appreciable ischaemic heart disease or cardiac failure. Patients who have had a recent myocardial infarct should have the operation postponed. Patients who have had a recent stroke should have endarterectomy delayed at least six weeks to allow cerebral autoregulation to recover and to reduce the perioperative chance of stroke. Patients with severe residual defects after major strokes will probably not derive any benefit from carotid surgery.

Conclusion

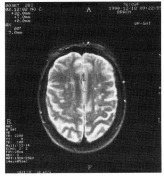

Magnetic resonance brain scan of patient with severe left internal carotid artery stenosis and moderate right sided stenosis. Note the larger number of areas of abnormal signal (small infarcts) on the side with more severe stenosis.

There is definitely a case for carotid endarterectomy in patients with more than 70% stenosis who have symptoms, but the benefit to other patients remains to be shown. The long term advantage of surgery in reducing risk of stroke to possibly 1% a year is offset by the operative risk. Patients who are unlikely to survive 12 months should not be offered surgery. Accurate audit of each surgeon's and anaesthetist's practice is imperative. If the combined morbidity and mortality exceeds 6% in a vascular centre, then it should not continue to practice carotid endarterectomy. The European and American carotid surgery trials continue to randomise patients with 30-70% stenosis. These trials will also provide more definite information about which patient subgroups are more likely to benefit from surgery and which are at most risk from the operation.

The results of carotid endarterectomy in asymptomatic carotid stenosis are awaited with interest.

RAYNAUD'S SYNDROME AND SIMILAR CONDITIONS

M H Grigg, John H N Wolfe

Raynaud's phenomenon

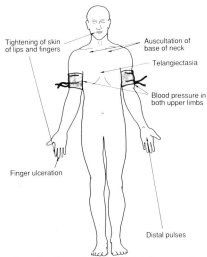

Examination of patients with Raynaud's phenomenon.

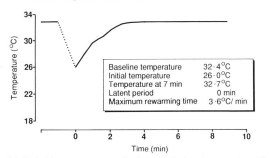

Digital skin temperature before and after immersion of hand in water at 20°C for one minute by a normal volunteer. Rewarming occurred within three minutes. Zero time is when the hand was removed from the water.

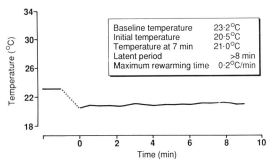

Digital skin temperature before and after immersion of hand in water at 20°C for one minute by a patient with Raynaud's phenomenon. Rewarming to baseline temperature had not occurred within nine minutes.

The circulation of the extremities can be regulated by temperature—for example, exposure to cold in a normal person will cause vasoconstriction and a decrease in blood flow to the skin. Abnormalities of this apparently simple response have been of interest since Maurice Raynaud described the syndrome that bears his name in 1862. He attributed the clinical signs that he observed to overactivity of the sympathetic nervous system, and so began a series of controversies that persist today.

Diagnosis

Underlying many of the controversies surrounding Raynaud's phenomenon is the subjectivity of the diagnosis. This depends on a history of the characteristic colour changes in the fingers that are provoked by exposure to cold, and—less reliably—by emotion; cold, however, is the only one of the factors that is universally accepted. These colour changes may be accompanied by parasthesia and other sensations, but pain is not a prominent feature.

Many tests have been devised to try to find an objective method of diagnosis. These include plethysmography (usually mercury in a silicone rubber strain gauge, which can monitor changes in the volume of the digit by arterial pulsation); Doppler ultrasonography (the digital arteries can be insonated to see if they are patent, and even to measure pressure); laser Doppler flowmetry and direct capillaroscopy (which can be used to assess the velocity of red blood cells in the microcirculation); and thermal entrainment (which measures changes in blood flow in one extremity while the other is exposed repeatedly to opposing thermal stimuli). Thermal entrainment is non-invasive, quick to do, and reproducible, and may be of most benefit in assessing the effects of drugs.

The simplest way of assessing skin blood flow is by measuring its temperature, as there is a linear relation between temperature and blood flow up to digital skin temperatures of 34°C. The absolute skin temperature is not, however, a good discriminator, because it is influenced by various factors (both internal and external) that are difficult to control. To separate normal from abnormal values it is necessary to apply a cold stimulus and then monitor rates of rewarming. Normal subjects rewarm rapidly after cessation of a mild cold stimulus (water at 20°C), whereas patients with Raynaud's phenomenon go through a latent period. In addition, once rewarming has begun patients with vaso-obstruction as well as vasospasm do not seem to rewarm as fast as normal subjects.

The idea that vessels "hyper-respond" to cold is attractive, but there has been a growing realisation that the pathophysiological defect is failure to recover from a cold stimulus rather than an initial over-response to it.

In 1893 Hutchinson drew attention to the association between Raynaud's phenomenon and scleroderma, and since that time the number of possible underlying disorders has increased. Although there is a need to separate the so called "primary" and "secondary" types, the distinction becomes more blurred as our understanding of the condition increases and "Raynaud's phenomenon" is seen as the final common pathway of a number of abnormalities. Initially secondary Raynaud's was thought to be uncommon, but with the search for an underlying disorder becoming more thorough this may not be the case.

Both vasospasm and fixed obstruction of the lumen of the digital vessels occur to a greater or lesser degree in most patients. More importantly there is concern that patients may progress from vasospasm to develop digital and microvascular obstruction. Undoubtedly this may be the result of progression of the underlying disease, but it could also be the result of continued, unprotected exposure to cold. The experience of patients who have had frostbite in the past and who subsequently develop hypersensitivity to cold in the affected part confirms that cold alone can cause severe damage.

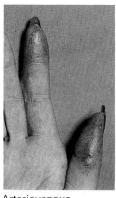

Arteriovenous malformation masquerading as Raynaud's phenomenon.

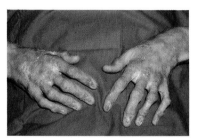

Hands showing severe scleroderma.

Incidence

The relative incidence of primary and secondary Raynaud's is entirely dependent on referral patterns. Thus more patients with secondary Raynaud's are seen in specialist Raynaud's clinics than in community practice.

The overall incidence of Raynaud's phenomenon, both primary and secondary, is difficult to estimate because of the lack of an objective method of diagnosis. Certainly about 90% of patients are women, and there is often a family history. Hypersensitivity to cold is common. In a study of female factory workers in Denmark the incidence was 22%, similar to that reported from the United States. Many patients have mild symptoms that begin when they are teenagers and gradually abate around the time of the menopause. Nevertheless, between 5% and 15% of patients with Raynaud's phenomenon will develop overt scleroderma (about 90% of patients with scleroderma also have Raynaud's phenomenon). Of most concern is the (fortunately) small group—less than 1%—who go on to develop digital gangrene and require amputation. Patients with poor prognoses cannot reliably be predicted in the early stages of their disease, but they do seem to develop vaso-obstruction in addition to vasospasm.

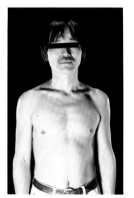

Patient with left cervical rib.

Clinical assessment

Having made the initial clinical diagnosis of Raynaud's phenomenon, the assessment should be directed at: (a) identifying any underlying disorders, and (b) assessing the effect of the disease on the patient, as this will indicate the treatment.

The patient should be questioned about family history, drug taking, and occupation—especially handling ice (as with some workers in the food industry) and the use of vibrating machinery. In addition, a history of arthralgia, dysphagia, or xerostomia should be sought as these suggest an underlying collagen disorder.

Physical examination should include careful assessment of upper limb pulses by both palpation and auscultation; the latter should be done over both the supraclavicular fossas and the deltopectoral triangle. These results, together with the measurements of blood pressure in both upper limbs, may show an anatomical distortion of the axillary or subclavian arteries—for example, as a result of cervical rib or band. Asymmetrical Raynaud's raises the possibility of a "mechanical," and therefore surgically correctable, arterial lesion. This is particularly true in the older age groups when atherosclerosis of the main upper limb arteries may be causing symptoms. A search should also be made for skin tightening, particularly of the fingers and around the mouth, for telangiectasia, and for carpal tunnel syndrome.

Investigations are to some extent determined by the suspicions aroused during clinical assessment, but should include full blood count, biochemical and urine analysis, and radiographs of the hands.

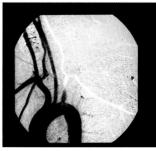

Digital subtraction angiogram showing subclavian "steal" syndrome.

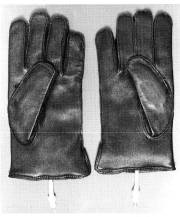

Vascutherm battery powered gloves.

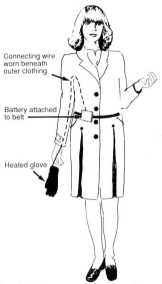

Connecting wire worn beneath outer clothing

Battery attached to belt

Heated glove

The glove is powered by a rechargable battery, and the connecting wire is inconspicuous beneath the clothing.

Other vasospastic conditions

Conditions with which Raynaud's phenomenon is associated

Connective tissue disorders:
  Scleroderma
  Systemic lupus erythematosus
  Rheumatoid arthritis
  Other

Obstructive arterial disease:
  Thoracic outlet syndrome
  Atherosclerosis
  Thromboangiitis obliterans

Occupations:
  Vibration
  Cold

Drugs:
  Ergotamine
  β-Blocking agents
  Cytotoxic agents
  Oral contraceptives

Miscellaneous:
  Neoplasia
  Neurological disorders
  Endocrinological disorders
  Arterial trauma
  Arteritis
  Other

Treatment

There is no cure for Raynaud's phenomenon. The palliative treatment must depend on the severity of the symptoms. For patients with mild symptoms explanation and reassurance may be all that is required. From the patient's point of view the problem is not only the "poor circulation," but also the anxiety that this provokes. If appropriate, community support may be given through the Raynaud's Association Trust, 112 Crewe Road, Alsager, Cheshire ST7 25A, telephone 0270-872776.

General advice is of paramount importance: stop smoking and avoid cold. Electrically heated gloves (Vascutherm) have been of great benefit to some patients. Skiers with this problem have found that the centrifugal force resulting from a windmill action of the arms can stave off the effects and maintain some perfusion of the finger tips.

For patients with moderate symptoms drugs may be needed. Thymoxamine (Opilon) is a mild α_1 and α_2 adrenergic receptor blocker that increases blood flow to the skin. In contrast with some other agents it has few side effects and is well tolerated in a dose of 40 mg four times a day. The calcium channel blocking agent nifedipine is also useful (maximum dose 20 mg twice a day); the patient should not be started on the full dose—an initial dose of 10 mg twice a day should be increased after a week to prevent side effects. For more resistant cases a combination of agents (to reduce the incidence of side effects)—for example, guanethidine 10 mg daily and prazosin 1 mg twice a day—may be considered.

The severe cases, particularly those in which there is ulceration or gangrene, are a challenge to the clinician. Admission to hospital may be required. Prostaglandin infusions, reserpine given intra-arterially, and plasmapheresis are all useful in some patients. Prostacyclin usually has a pleasing immediate result and in some patients the improvement may be maintained for several months. Two or three admissions to hospital for infusions can tide a patient over the bleak winter months. The patient is started on 6 ng/kg/hour and the dose increased to 15 ng/kg/hour depending on the effect and the side effects. Side effects are dose related, and almost immediate relief will be obtained by reducing the infusion.

The indications for cervicothoracic sympathectomy are few. Beneficial effects, especially in patients with connective tissue disorders, are difficult to achieve and are short lived.

Acrocyanosis may be difficult to distinguish from Raynaud's phenomenon, but as the management is similar the distinction may not be of critical importance. The absence of temporal fluctuation of symptoms together with the presence of oedema may assist the diagnosis.

White finger syndrome is an occupational disease. Sustained exposure to vibration at given frequencies results in permanent neurological and musculoskeletal changes.

Livedo reticularis is primarily a cosmetic problem confined to the legs. The cause seems to be spasm of the cutaneous arterioles, which become more prominent when they are cold. The inadequacy of drug treatment has in the past led to treatment with lumbar sympathectomy, with mixed results.

Erythromelalgia and causalgia—Whereas pain is not a feature of Raynaud's disease, burning pain of the hands or feet suggests erythromelalgia. In many respects this is the opposite of Raynaud's, because heat provokes an attack and the patient seeks relief with cold water or by standing barefoot on a cold floor. β Blocking agents have been used to obtain symptomatic relief; carbamazepine 200 mg twice a day may also be beneficial. Burning pain is also a feature of causalgia, in which the association with previous sensory nerve damage is well established. There is often a functional element as well.

Chilblains—Patients prone to chilblains complain bitterly of the cold. This is an inflammatory condition—in chronic cases there is angiitis with intimal proliferation and a perivascular infiltrate of neutrophils and lymphocytes. Protection from the cold, anti-Raynaud's drugs, and anti-inflammatory ointments may be helpful.

Other causes of digital gangrene

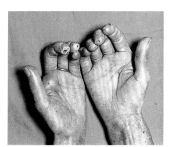

Severe Raynaud's phenomenon can result in ulceration of the finger tips.

Digital ulceration or gangrene may also be caused by non-vasospastic conditions. Emboli may be discharged from the fibrillating atrium, the ventricle after a myocardial infarction, or from an aneurysm of the subclavian artery. Arteriovenous malformations in the hand can cause enough shunting of blood to result in distal ischaemia. Occasionally, thrombotic disorders such as polycythaemia or thrombocythaemia may cause digital ischaemia, but this is most unusual in the hand.

Vascutherm gloves are distributed by Camp Ltd, Staple Gardens, Northgate House, Winchester SO23 8ST, telephone: 0962-55248.

PERIPHERAL ARTERIOVENOUS MALFORMATIONS

D J Allison, Anne Kennedy

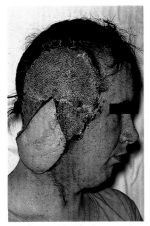

A young patient with life threatening arteriovenous malformation of right ear and scalp. This was treated by preoperative embolisation, which made excision possible. The carotid artery was used as the base of the pedicle for a free flap transfer. The patient survived as a result of cooperation between radiologist, vascular surgeon, and plastic surgeon.

The term arteriovenous malformation encompasses a bewildering variety of lesions, many of which are rarely treated outside specialist units. The lesions can occur anywhere in the body and the symptoms and signs depend on the site, size, and degree of shunting through the lesion. Their aetiology is uncertain. Some are clearly post-traumatic and some are congenital; others appear years after birth, possibly in relation to either accidental or iatrogenic trauma. Much work is in progress to try to isolate an "angiogenesis factor" that will clarify their pathophysiology.

Classification of the lesions is difficult because of the plethora of descriptive terms used by both clinicians and pathologists. At angiography, however, most lesions can be classified by their flow characteristics into one of three groups:

Group 1—Predominantly arterial or arteriovenous lesions
Group 2—Lesions affecting tiny vessels including capillaries
Group 3—Predominantly venous lesions.

This is a classification on which therapeutic decisions can be based, though it does not necessarily bear any accurate relation to the histological appearances of the lesions. This article is confined to benign lesions.

History

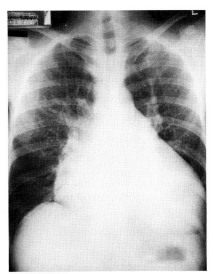

Chest radiograph showing massive cardiomegaly that occurs with high output cardiac failure.

Group 1 lesions produce most symptoms and have appreciable associated mortality; those in group 2 tend to cause cosmetic problems; and group 3 lesions may cause troublesome local aching but rarely produce severe symptoms.

Group 1

The most common symptoms of group 1 lesions are pain, increase in the size of the limb or digit, venous hypertension, distal ischaemia, recurrent bleeding, and deformity. When they occur in the head and neck tinnitus can be a serious problem, and difficulties in breathing and speech occur when the tongue is enlarged. Large group 1 lesions can also cause cardiac failure secondary to the considerable decrease in venous return; symptoms such as undue tiredness and dyspnoea on exertion must always be sought.

Group 2

In group 2 lesions the presenting complaint is usually cosmetic, such as a "port wine stain." Some lesions can, however, cause bleeding—for example, epistaxis in patients with hereditary haemorrhagic telangiectasia or gastrointestinal haemorrhage in patients with colonic angiodysplasia. In patients with the Sturge-Weber syndrome (capillary naevus of the upper face associated with underlying vascular abnormalities of the ipsilateral leptomeninges and choroid plexus) there may be progressive degeneration and atrophy of the affected cerebral hemisphere.

Group 3

The principal complaints of patients with group 3 lesions are usually about the appearance of the area, but local oedema, pain, and venous ulceration can cause considerable discomfort. All patients should be questioned about family history and previous trauma as some arteriovenous malformations are activated by local trauma (including dental surgery) and some may be post-traumatic arteriovenous fistulas.

Examination

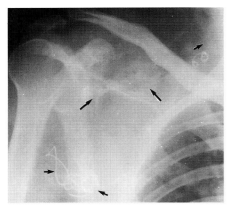

Radiograph of right shoulder showing extensive group 1 arteriovenous malformation that has caused pronounced bone destruction (arrowed). Note the multiple embolisation coils (arrow heads).

Group 1

Group 1 arteriovenous malformations present as pulsatile swellings with bruits. They may cause disfigurement, local pressure effects, trophic changes, local venous hypertension, deformity, gigantism, bone destruction, distal ischaemia, haemorrhage, and an increase in cardiac output—ultimately causing cardiac failure in some patients.

Branham's sign may be elicited in some patients with group 1 arteriovenous malformations. When there is an appreciable shunt, temporary occlusion of that shunt by occlusion of the proximal artery (for example, the femoral artery) will result in reflexive slowing of the heart.

In *Allen's test* the radial and ulnar arteries are occluded at the wrist and the hand is exercised. The arteries are then released one at a time to establish which is the dominant feeding vessel.

Group 2

Some group 2 lesions may not be apparent on clinical examination—for example, angiodysplasia of the colon. Superficial skin lesions appear as port wine stains, and patients who complain of epistaxis may have telangiectasia visible on the skin or nasal mucosa.

Group 3

Group 3 lesions usually present as non-pulsatile swellings that are easily emptied by compression, fill by gravity, and—when superficial—cause blue discolouration of the overlying skin.

Investigation

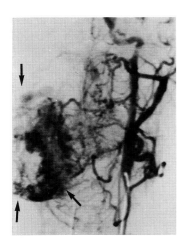

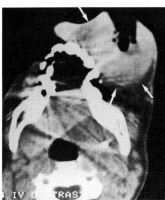

Group 1 arteriovenous malformation of right cheek. Digital subtraction angiogram (top) shows large, ulcerated, vascular mass. Computed tomogram (bottom) shows full extent of lesion (arrowed) before plastic surgery. The lesion had been quiescent until the patient became pregnant.

Many arteriovenous malformations do not require special investigation; the temptation to feel that something must be done and therefore to send the patient for radiological examination should be resisted. Angiography should be requested only if the result is likely to influence the management of the patient, and other methods of investigation may be more appropriate initially. Plain radiographs may show phleboliths and bone destruction; venography, Doppler ultrasonography, computed tomography, and magnetic resonance imaging may show the extent of the lesion and its precise relation with surrounding structures.

Group 1

Group 1 lesions typically have enlarged feeding arteries and prominent draining veins, and the degree of arteriovenous shunting depends on the size and number of abnormal communications between the arteries and veins. Characteristically there is fast flow through the arteries, early or immediate venous filling, and rapid clearing of contrast medium. In acquired arteriovenous fistulas venous filling is almost immediate as a result of the relatively wide and localised arteriovenous communication.

If angiography is used large volumes of contrast medium injected at high pressure by automatic pumps may be necessary to ensure adequate opacification. Limb tourniquets or balloon occlusion catheters slow down the flow through the lesions, and rapid sequence filming on digital subtraction angiography or 105 mm film is essential to define their anatomy.

Group 2

Angiography is rarely indicated for the small vessels affected in group 2 lesions, except in patients with epistaxis or gastrointestinal bleeding who are going to be treated by embolisation or operation.

Group 3

In this group of patients it may be important to exclude an arterial element to the vascular malformation, but usually arteriography has no place. Venography shows the dilated serpentine veins, but many of these do not fill, so its role is limited. Computed tomography or magnetic resonance imaging may play a part by identifying those well defined lesions with localised limits that could be excised, but most are diffuse so that surgical interference would be meddlesome.

Management

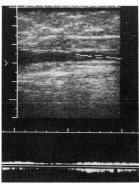

Doppler ultrasonograph showing patent deep veins in association with an extensive venous malformation of the lower limb.

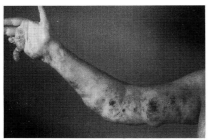

An extensive disfiguring lesion that was not amenable to treatment by embolisation.

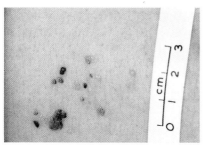

Lymphangioma, the extent of which was far greater than indicated by surface lesions.

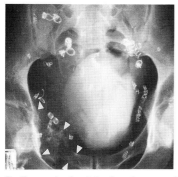

Radiograph of pelvis showing massive group 1 arteriovenous malformation that required more than 17 embolisations to control it. Note multiple embolisation coils and also destruction of right ischium and pubis.

Arteriovenous malformations should always be managed jointly by a vascular surgeon and an interventional radiologist with experience in embolisation.

Group 1

Embolisation is the treatment of choice for group 1 lesions if it is technically possible. The exception is when the communication is wide and short—for example, in acquired arteriovenous fistulas in which the risk of pulmonary embolism is such that operation should be preferred. Far too many patients are operated on first, and then referred to a radiologist when this has failed. Ligation of the main feeding arteries can be a disaster as any revascularisation of the arteriovenous malformation is likely to originate from smaller more inaccessible vessels, making subsequent embolisation difficult if not impossible. For some lesions embolisation may precede operation, which will be done when the vascularity of the lesion has been decreased. This is particularly important when the histological appearance of the lesion is in question.

Group 2

Group 2 lesions are embolised only occasionally, but some superficial lesions may respond to laser treatment and all patients should be referred for cosmetic advice—particularly those whose faces are affected. Extensive lymphangiomas may weep lymph persistently so that excision may be beneficial, but the skin lesions are usually the tip of the iceberg and the subcutaneous lesion may be much more extensive than first thought.

Group 3

Group 3 lesions are best managed conservatively (or occasionally by operation). The presence of a localised superficial venous network may tempt the surgeon to intervene, but usually the lesion is infiltrating the underlying muscle, so early recurrence is common.

Embolisation

Successful embolisation entails blocking the feeding arteries as close to the lesion as possible, and blocking its nidus to decrease the likelihood of recanalisation. The main access vessels should be left patent to permit further treatment. Vessels supplying normal neighbouring structures should not be touched, and the breaking off of small emboli into the circulation, through which they may pass to the lungs, must be avoided.

When the malformation is in a vital organ (such as kidney or liver) a decision may have to be made about whether eradication of the malformation is more important than the preservation of some function of that organ. Embolisation outside the central nervous system is usually safe with low morbidity, but because inadvertent embolisation of normal vessels within the central nervous system could have disastrous consequences any embolisation within the central nervous system should be done only by experienced neuroradiologists.

In most cases embolisation is palliative rather than curative. Several procedures may be required to bring a large arteriovenous malformation under "control" and the patient must be followed up in the outpatient clinic (or by the general practitioner) with a view to re-embolisation as and when necessary.

Group 1 arteriovenous malformations are particularly likely to worsen during pregnancy, and both doctor and patient should be aware of this as it may affect the timing of embolisation, or pregnancy, or both.

Conclusions

Patients with arteriovenous malformations should always be assessed by a vascular surgeon together with an experienced interventional radiologist

Arteriovenous malformations are best managed in specialist centres, the patient being assessed jointly by a vascular surgeon and an interventional radiologist.

Lesions can usually be classified clinically into groups 1, 2, and 3; if there is doubt a Doppler ultrasound examination will differentiate group 1 lesions from group 2 and group 3 lesions.

Arteriovenous malformations cause disfigurement, discomfort, and danger to many patients. The development of effective techniques of embolisation during the past two decades means that we can now offer

Complications of embolism

- Postembolisation syndrome:
  Malaise
  Fever
  Pain
  Leucocytosis
- Specific to embolisation:
  Tissue ischaemia
  Tissue breakdown
  Sepsis
  Inadvertent embolisation of normal
      tissue
- Related to angiography:
  Renal failure
  Vessel dissection
  Reaction to contrast medium
  Reaction to anaesthetic

treatment to some patients for whom none was possible previously.

Interventional radiology is developing fast. New techniques, equipment, and embolic agents are continually being introduced. It may soon be possible safely to embolise group 3 lesions percutaneously or from the venous side. In addition, work is progressing on instruments through which direct laser destruction of vascular endothelium will be possible.

Whatever new developments arise the key to safe and effective treatment of arteriovenous malformations is the closest possible cooperation between clinician and radiologist. In particular, surgical ligation of the main feeding arteries as an alternative to complete surgical excision must be avoided at all costs as this may preclude subsequent embolisation.

The lymphangioma was prepared by the audiovisual department, St Mary's Hospital, London, and the remaining illustrations were prepared by Westway Graphics, Hammersmith Hospital, London.

INDEX

Index

Index